Rapid Surgery

Second Edition

Cara R. Baker
Surgical Registrar
UK

George Reese
Surgical Registrar
UK

James T.H. Teo
Charing Cross Hospital
UK

WILEY-BLACKWELL

A John Wiley & Sons, Ltd., Publication

This edition first published 2010, © 2010 by Cara R Baker, James T H Teo and George Reese
Previous edition: 2005

Blackwell Publishing was acquired by John Wiley & Sons in February 2007. Blackwells publishing program has been merged with Wileys global Scientific, Technical and Medical business to form Wiley-Blackwell.

Registered office: John Wiley & Sons Ltd, The Atrium, Southern Gate, Chichester, West Sussex, PO19 8SQ, UK

Editorial offices: 9600 Garsington Road, Oxford, OX4 2DQ, UK
The Atrium, Southern Gate, Chichester, West Sussex, PO19 8SQ, UK
111 River Street, Hoboken, NJ 07030-5774, USA

For details of our global editorial offices, for customer services and for information about how to apply for permission to reuse the copyright material in this book please see our website at www.wiley.com/wiley-blackwell

Library of Congress Cataloging-in-Publication Data

Baker, Cara R.
  Rapid surgery / Cara R. Baker, James T.H. Teo, George Reese. – 2nd ed.
    p. ; cm. – (Rapid series)
  Rev. ed. of: Rapid surgery / Ebube E. Obi ... [et al.] ; editorial advisor, Brian Davidson. 2005.
  Includes bibliographical references.
  ISBN 978-1-4051-9329-0
  1. Surgery–Handbooks, manuals, etc. I. Teo, James T. H. II. Reese, George, Dr. III. Rapid surgery. IV. Title. V. Series: Rapid series.
  [DNLM: 1. General Surgery–Handbooks. WO 39 B167r 2010]
  RD37.R375 2010
  617–dc22

                                                                                    2010008344

ISBN: 9781405193290

A catalogue record for this book is available from the British Library.

Set in 7.5/9.5pt Frutiger-Light by Thomson Digital, Noida, India.
Printed and bound in Malaysia by Vivar Printing Sdn Bhd

1   2010

Rapid S...

Contents

Head and neck surgery

Hepatobiliary surgery

Lower gastrointestinal surgery

Neurosurgery

Opthalmology

Orthopaedic surgery

Plastic surgery

Procedures

Upper gastrointestinal surgery

Urology

Vascular surgery

Preface

In *Rapid Surgery*, we envisaged a student revision aid that focused on key facts presented in a classical mnemonic format to facilitate learning. This consisted of each subject presented in the subheadings of D: Definition; A: Aetiology; A: Associations/Risk Factors; E: Epidemiology; H: History; E: Examination; P: Pathology/Pathogenesis; I: Investigations; M: Management; C: Complications and P: Prognosis. In this second edition, the presentation has been revised with clearer subheadings to help the reader. We have updated the content and introduced new topics, for example, bariatric surgery, that have an important place in modern surgical practice.

We hope that this book will continue to compliment your personal and ward-based learning and you enjoy reading it.

We thank our previous contributors, Dr Mark Teo, Dr Ebube Obi and Professor Brian Davidson, MD, FRCS. We thank our teachers through the years, Wiley-Blackwell publishing for their support and the patients who were our chief educators.

Finally, we would like to acknowledge our families for their support, especially the Bakers and Ping Lim.

Cara R. Baker
George Reese
James T.H. Teo

List of abbreviations

AAA	abdominal aortic aneurysm
ABC	airway, breathing, circulation
ABG	arterial blood gas
ABPI	ankle–brachial pressure index
ACAG	acute closed-angle glaucoma
ACE	angiotensin-converting enzyme
ACTH	adrenocorticotropic hormone
AKA	above-knee amputation
AMI	acute myocardial infarction
ANDI	aberrations of normal development and involution
AP	anterioposterior
ARDS	acute respiratory distress syndrome
ASA	American Society of Anesthesiologists
5-ASA	5-aminosalicylic acid
ATLS	advanced trauma life support
AV	arteriovenous
AVM	arteriovenous malformation
AXR	abdominal X-ray
BCG	bacillus Calmette–Guérin
BP	blood pressure
BPH	benign prostatic hyperplasia
CABG	coronary artery bypass grafting
CAVATAS	Carotid and Vertebral Artery Transluminal Angioplasty Study
CEA	carcinoembryonic antigen
CMV	cytomegalovirus
CRP	C-reactive protein
CSDH	chronic subdural haematoma
CT	computed tomography
CVA	cerebrovascular accident
CVP	central venous pressure
CXR	chest X-ray
DM	diabetes mellitus
DMSA	dimercaptosuccinic acid
DNA	deoxyribonucleic acid
DTPA	diethylenetriamine pentaacetic acid
DVT	deep vein thrombosis
EBV	Epstein–Barr virus
ECG	electrocardiogram
ECST	European Carotid Surgery Trial
EEG	electroencephalogram/graphy
ERCP	endoscopic retrograde cholangiopancreatography
EVAR	endovascular aortic aneurysm repair
FAP	familial adenomatous polyposis
FBC	full blood count
FEV	forced expiratory volume
FFP	fresh frozen plasma
FNA	fine-needle aspiration
FNAC	fine-needle aspiration cytology
G&S	group and save
GCS	Glasgow Coma Scale

GI	gastrointestinal
GIST	gastrointestinal stromal tumour
GORD	gastro-oesophageal reflux disease
HCC	hepatocellular carcinoma
HCG	human chorionic gonadotropin
HDU	high dependency unit
HIV	human immunodeficiency virus
HNPCC	hereditary nonpolyposis colorectal cancer
HPFs	high power fields
HRT	hormone replacement therapy
IBD	inflammatory bowel disease
IC	inspiratory capacity
ICP	intracranial pressure
IgG	immunoglobulin G
INR	international normalized ratio
IOP	intraocular pressure
IPSS	International Prostate Symptom Score
ITU	intensive therapy unit
IV	intravenous
IVC	inferior vena cava
IVU	intravenous urogram
JVP	jugular venous pressure
KUB	kidney, ureter, bladder
LBO	large-bowel obstruction
LDH	lactate dehydrogenase
LFT	liver function test
LHRH	luteinising hormone–releasing hormone
LIF	left iliac fossa
LMN	lower motor neuron
LUTS	lower urinary tract symptom
MALT	mucosa-associated lymphoid tissue
MC&S	microscopy culture and sensitivity
MEN	multiple endocrine neoplasia
MI	myocardial infarction
MRA	magnetic resonance angiography
MRI	magnetic resonance imaging
MRCP	magnetic resonance cholangiopancreatography
MSU	midstream urine
MTP	metatarsophalangeal
M-VAC	methotrexate, vinblastine, doxorubicin and cisplatin
NASCET	North American Symptomatic Carotid Endarterectomy Trial
NCAM	neural cell adhesion molecule
NG	nasogastric
NPI	Nottingham Prognostic Index
OCP	oral contraceptive pill
OGD	oesophagogastroduodenoscopy
pANCA	p antineutrophil cytoplasmic autoantibody
PBC	primary biliary cirrhosis
PE	pulmonary embolism
PET	positron emission tomography
POAG	primary open-angle glaucoma
PPI	proton pump inhibitor
PR	per rectum
PSA	prostate-specific antigen

PSC	primary sclerosing cholangitis
PTC	percutaneous transhepatic cholangiography
PTFE	polytetrafluoroethylene
PUFA	polyunsaturated fatty acid
PUVA	psoralen ultraviolet A
RAS	renal artery stenosis
RBBB	right bundle branch block
RBC	red blood cell
RCC	renal cell carcinoma
RIF	right iliac fossa
RPE	retinal pigment epithelium
SBO	small-bowel obstruction
SBP	spontaneous bacterial peritonitis
SC	subcutaneous
SDH	subdural haematoma
SFJ	saphenofemoral junction
SIADH	syndrome of inappropriate antidiuretic hormone
SLE	systemic lupus erythematosus
spp.	species (pl)
ST	sinus tachycardia
SVC	superior vena cava
TB	tuberculosis
TED	thrombo-embolic deterrent
TIA	transient ischaemic attack
TNM	tumour, node, metastasis
tPA	tissue-plasminogen activator
TRUS	transrectal ultrasonography
TURBT	trans-urethral resection of bladder tumour
TURP	trans-urethral resection of prostate
U&E	urea and electrolytes
UICC	International Union Against Cancer
UMN	upper motor neuron
URTI	upper respiratory tract infection
USG	ultrasonography
USS	ultrasound scan
UTI	urinary tract infection
UV	ultraviolet
WCC	white cell count

Breast abscess

DEFINITION
Localised infection with pus collection in breast tissue. The two main forms are puerperal (lactational) and non-puerperal.

AETIOLOGY
Lactational: Milk stasis associated with infection, most commonly with *Staphylococcus aureus*, coagulase-negative staphylococci.

Non-puerperal: *S. aureus* and anaerobes, often enterococci or *Bacteroides* spp. (TB and actinomycosis are rare causes). Smoking, mammary duct ectasia/periductal mastitis, associated inflammatory breast cancer should be excluded. Also associated with wound infections after breast surgery, diabetes and steroid therapy.

EPIDEMIOLOGY
Lactational breast abscesses are common and tend to occur soon after starting breast-feeding and on weaning, when incomplete emptying of the breast results in stasis and engorgement. Non-lactational abscesses are more common in those aged 30–60 years and in smokers.

HISTORY
The patient complains of discomfort and development of a painful swelling in an area of the breast. She may complain of feeling unwell and feverish.

Women with a non-puerperal abscess often have a history of previous infections, systemic upset is often less pronounced.

EXAMINATION
Local: The area of the breast is swollen, warm and tender. The overlying skin may be inflamed; examination of the nipple may reveal cracks or fissures. In non-puerperal cases, there may be evidence of scars or tissue distortion from previous episodes, or signs of duct ectasia, e.g. nipple retraction.

Systemic: Pyrexia, tachycardia.

INVESTIGATIONS
Imaging: Ultrasound + aspiration for microscopy, culture and sensitivity of pus samples.

MANAGEMENT
Medical: Early, cellulitic phase may be treated with antibiotics (flucloxacillin in the case of lactational, with the addition of metronidazole in non-puerperal abscesses). Regular breast drainage to prevent milk stasis.

Surgical: *Lactational*: Daily needle aspiration with antibiotic cover may be successful. Formal incision and drainage is reserved for larger abscesses (>5 cm). The incision should allow full drainage and be cosmetically acceptable; loculi are explored and broken down. The wound may be packed lightly and left open, with daily packing, or primary closure performed. Breastfeeding should continue from the non-affected breast and the affected side emptied either manually or with a breast pump. Advice on avoiding cracked nipples.

Non-puerperal: Open drainage should be avoided, or carried out through a small incision. Definitive treatment should be carried out once the infection has settled by the excision of the involved duct system.

COMPLICATIONS
Slow wound healing, difficulties in breastfeeding, poor cosmetic outcome and mammary fistula formation; rarely, overlying skin undergoes necrosis.

PROGNOSIS
If untreated, a breast abscess will eventually point and spontaneously discharge onto the skin surface. Non-puerperal abscesses tend to recur.

Breast cancer

DEFINITION
Malignancy arising from breast tissue.

AETIOLOGY
Combination of genetic and environmental factors.

Genetics: Most cases are polygenic risk with 5–10% attributable to inherited factors. BRCA-1 (17q) and BRCA-2 (13q) gene mutations are implicated in ~2% of cases (carriers have lifetime risk up to 87%). Rare genetic breast cancer syndromes include Li–Fraumeni syndrome (TP53), Cowden's syndrome (PTEN), Peutz–Jeghers syndrome (STK11/LKB1), ataxia-telagiectasia (ATM) and Muir–Torre syndrome (MSH2/MLH1).

ASSOCIATIONS/RISK FACTORS
Age, prolonged exposure to female sex hormones (particularly oestrogen), nulliparity, early menarche, late menopause, menopausal hormone replacement therapy, obesity, alcohol.

EPIDEMIOLOGY
Worldwide, the leading cause of cancer death in women (second only to lung cancer in the USA). The lifetime risk is 1 : 9 in the UK. Peak incidence in 40- to 70-year-olds. Rare in men (<1% of all breast cancers).

HISTORY
May be detected from screening.
Symptoms of primary: Breast lump (usually painless), changes in breast shape, nipple discharge.
Symptoms of secondary spread: Axillary lump, bone pain, weight loss, paraneoplastic syndromes (e.g. cerebellar syndrome).

EXAMINATION
Inspection of breasts with the patient upright and supine, assessing for asymmetry, peau d'orange appearance of skin (oedema), dimpling or tethering, nipple scaling or inversion or, in advanced cases, ulceration.
Palpation using clockwise radial technique (for hard, irregular, fixed lumps).
Examination for palpable axillary, supraclavicular lymph nodes, chest abnormalities, hepatomegaly, bony tenderness.

INVESTIGATIONS
Triple assessment: Standardised approach to investigating a breast lump, consisting of clinical examination, imaging (mammography, ultrasound, MRI) and tissue diagnosis (cytology or biopsy).
Mammogram (Fig. 1): Useful screening investigation in women >35 years. In the UK, screening begins after the age of 50. Standard views are craniocaudal and mediolateral oblique. Features of malignancy include branching or linear microcalcifications and spiculated lesions.
Ultrasound: To identify benign cystic lesions from sinister solid lesions. More useful in women <35 years.
Fine-needle aspiration: Minimally invasive, allows cytology of discrete breast lumps and drainage of cysts.
Core biopsy: Can be image guided, enables histological diagnosis.
Sentinal lymph node biopsy: Radioactive tracer and/or blue dye is injected near the breast lesion, and a nuclear scan identifies the sentinel node and the node is biopsied to detect spread.
Staging: CT (chest, abdomen, pelvis), PET or bone scanning for metastases.
Blood: FBC, U&Es, Ca^{2+}, bone profile, LFT, tumour marker (CA-15-3).

Breast cancer (continued)

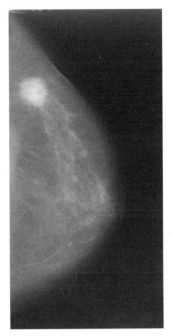

Figure 1 Mammogram showing a spiculated breast cancer lesion.

Histology:

- *In situ carcinoma*: Non-invasive with basement membrane intact – ductal or lobular carcinoma in situ (DCIS, LCIS).
- *Invasive*: Most common is ductal carcinoma (75% of breast cancers).
- *Others*: Lobular (10–15%, 'Indian filing' arrangement of cells), tubular, mucinous, medullary, cribriform, papillary and Paget's disease of the nipple (ductal carcinoma *in situ* infiltrating the nipple).
- *Phlloides*: Fibroepithelial tumours that can be benign or malignant.
- *Molecular prognostic factors*: Oestrogen and progesterone receptors (ER, PR) and HER-2 expression (20–30% of cancers) are valuable prognostic indicators and guide treatment. Flow cytometry measures DNA content (ploidy) and S-phase fraction (cell proliferation rate).

Grading: The Nottingham modification of the Bloom and Richardson grading system is a prognostic indicator. Three features assessed are tubule formation, nuclear size/pleomorphism and number of mitoses. Scores are used to generate Grades 1 (well differentiated) to 3 (poorly differentiated).

Staging: The UICC TNM-staging system.

Tumour size (T): T1: <2 cm; T2: 2–5 cm; T3: >5 cm; T4: any size with chest wall or skin extension.

Nodes (N): N1: mobile ipsilateral axillary; N2: fixed ipsilateral axillary; N3: ipsilateral internal mammary nodes.

Metastases (M): M0: no distant metastases; M1: distant metastases.

Breast cancer (continued)

MANAGEMENT

Multidisciplinary management: Includes breast surgeon, radiologist, oncologist and breast care nurses. Surgery to remove the cancer depends on the size, location, type, stage and consideration of the individual patient's wishes.

Breast-conserving surgery: Wide local excision/segmental mastectomy (single cancer, <5 cm, can be excised as a whole and patient is willing to undergo radiotherapy). Smaller lesions may need radiological wire localisation.

Modified radical mastectomy: Total mastectomy, axillary lymph node dissection.

Axillary surgery: Is necessary for node staging and ranges from sentinel node biopsy (on average three nodes removed) to level III clearance (lymph nodes up to and above pectoralis minor muscle).

Breast reconstruction: Often as a delayed procedure, occasionally concurrently with surgical excision. Breast prostheses, latissimus dorsi or transverse rectus abdominis myocutaneous flaps are methods used.

Radiotherapy: External beam radiotherapy following breast-conserving surgery, occasionally as neoadjuvent therapy and in palliation of advanced tumours.

Chemotherapy: Treatment can be in neoadjuvent, adjuvant and palliative settings. More often in premenopausal women, rapidly progressive disease, visceral involvement, oestrogen receptor-negative tumours or where hormonal treatment has failed. Combination regimens, e.g. cyclophosphamide, methotrexate and 5-fluorouracil (CMF), are tailored to the individual patient.

Hormonal therapy: Includes selective oestrogen receptor modulators, e.g. tamoxifen, the main first-line therapy for oestrogen receptor-positive tumours. Others include aromatase inhibitors in postmenopausal women, e.g. anastrozole or letrozole; ovarian ablation with LHRH-analogues, e.g. goserelin; and selective oestrogen receptor downregulators, e.g. fulvestrant and progestins.

Biological therapy: Trastuzumab (Herceptin) is a monoclonal antibody against HER-2 receptor (cell growth promoter) used in combination with chemotherapy in node and HER-2-positive cancer, and is shown to improve disease-free and overall survival.

COMPLICATIONS

Significant psychological morbidity from diagnosis or physical deformity from surgery. Metastases can cause bone pain, hypercalcaemia, cord compression and cerebral, abdominal or pulmonary complications.

From tamoxifen: Endometrial cancer, venous thrombosis. Aromatase inhibitors: joint/muscle ache, osteoporosis. Herceptin: cardiotoxicity.

From surgery: Wound infection, haematoma, lymphoedema, shoulder pain, sensory loss (the intercostobrachial nerve is commonly sacrificed, resulting in an area of numbness on the inner, upper arm), local recurrence.

From radiotherapy: Fatigue, skin changes, lymphoedema.

PROGNOSIS

Depends on type, grade and stage. Overall 5-year survival 100% if localised to breast, 50–90% for node-positive disease and 20% with distant metastases.

Breast disease, benign

DEFINITION
Non-malignant conditions of the breast, including physiopathological lesions of epithelial, stromal, fat or vascular components of the breast.

Fibroadenoma: Result from hyperplasia of a breast lobule and contain both normal epithelial and connective tissue elements.

Fat necrosis: Irregular and necrotic adipocytes, amorphous material and inflammatory cells, including foreign body giant cells, can mimic malignancy.

Sclerosing adenosis: Is an aberration of normal involution.

Duct ectasia: Occurs when central ducts become dilated with duct secretions; if leakage occurs into periductal tissue, this causes an inflammatory reaction (periductal mastitis).

AETIOLOGY
Breast tissue undergoes a wide range of changes under endocrine control. Fat necrosis occurs secondary to trauma. The ANDI (aberrations of normal development and involution) classification maps benign conditions according to both the pathogenesis and the degree of abnormality. Please see **Associations/Risk Factors**.

ASSOCIATIONS/RISK FACTORS
May be less common in those on contraceptive pill. Smoking is a risk factor for periductal mastitis.

EPIDEMIOLOGY
Commonly estimated only 10–20% of cases come to histological diagnosis. Diffuse fibrocystic changes are very common, seen in as many as 60% of women, and 70% experience mastalgia. Fibroadenomas are more common in the 15–25 age group, breast cysts in 40- to 50-year-olds, and usually disappear after menopause unless on hormone replacement therapy (HRT).

HISTORY
History of breast discomfort or pain (cyclical or non-cyclical mastalgia), swelling or lump. Nipple discharge (if bloodstained, malignancy should be suspected). Risk factors for breast cancer should be ascertained, including family history, menstrual history, pregnancies, use of OCP or hormone replacement therapy.

EXAMINATION
Focal or diffuse nodularity of breasts.

Fibroadenomas are usually smooth, well-circumscribed and mobile lumps (1–2 cm in diameter, 'breast mouse').

Yellow/green nipple discharge (duct ectasia).

Features of malignancy are absent, e.g. dimpling, peau d'orange skin changes, enlarged axillary lymph nodes.

INVESTIGATIONS
Usually performed in the context of triple assessment:
1. Clinical examination.
2. Imaging: Mammography (craniocaudal and oblique mediolateral views ± spot compression and magnification views) or USS in younger patients (<35 years). Benign masses are less likely to be calcified (microcalcifications are highly suggestive of malignancy). MRI scanning can also be useful.
3. Cytology/histology: By FNA (fine-needle aspiration) cytology or trucut or excision biopsy.

MANAGEMENT
Conservative: Symptomatic treatment, e.g. analgesia, evening primrose oil (a rich source of gammalinoleic acid) for mastalgia. Advice on wearing supportive bra and diet (reduced dietary fat). Danazol is used as second-line treatment. (17-α-ethinyl testosterone suppresses gonadotropin secretion, prevents LH surge and inhibits ovarian steroid formation). Fibroadenomas may be treated conservatively or removed if large or on request.

Breast disease, benign (continued)

Simple cysts do not need aspiration unless clinically indicated and, on aspiration, should disappear completely. If not, it should be treated as a breast lump.

Surgery: Includes removal or excision biopsy of breast lump; a wide local excision should be performed if there is any suspicion that it is not benign. Microdochectomy is performed for intraductal papillomas. Hadfield's (or Adair's) operation excises central ducts in duct ectasia.

COMPLICATIONS

Pain, recurrence.

PROGNOSIS

Good, although recurrence is common. Fibroadenomas: no increased risk of cancer in woman with simple FA and no increased family history of breast cancer.

Lung cancer

DEFINITION

Primary malignant neoplasm of the lung. WHO classification of bronchocarcinoma: small cell (20%) and non-small cell (80%) – squamous cell carcinoma, adenocarcinoma, large-cell carcinoma, adenosquamous carcinoma.

AETIOLOGY

Primary lung tumours: Factors such as smoking (active or passive) and asbestos exposure are thought to ultimately cause genetic mutations that result in neoplastic transformation. Tumours generally arise in main or lobar bronchi (see Fig. 2), and adenocarcinomas tend to occur more peripherally.

Secondary tumours: The lung is a common site for metastasis (see Fig. 3).

ASSOCIATIONS/RISK FACTORS

Smoking, occupational exposures (polycyclic hydrocarbons, asbestos, nickel, chromium, cadmium, radon), atmospheric pollution.

EPIDEMIOLOGY

Most common fatal malignancy in the West (18% of cancer mortality worldwide), 35,000 deaths per year (UK), 3× more common in men (but ↑ in women).

HISTORY

May be asymptomatic with radiographic abnormality (5%).

Due to primary: Cough, haemoptysis, chest pain, recurrent pneumonia.

Due to local invasion: For example, brachial plexus (Pancoast's tumour) causing pain in the shoulder or arm, left recurrent laryngeal nerve leading to hoarseness and bovine cough, oesophagus (dysphagia), palpitations (arrhythmias).

Due to metastatic disease or paraneoplastic phenomena: Weight loss, fatigue, bone pain or fractures, fits.

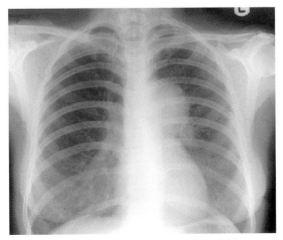

Figure 2 Chest radiograph showing primary bronchial carcinoma behind left hilum.

Lung cancer (continued)

EXAMINATION

There may be no signs.

Fixed monophonic wheeze.

Signs of lobar collapse or pleural effusion.

Signs of metastases (e.g. supraclavicular lymphadenopathy or hepatomegaly).

Horner's syndrome.

INVESTIGATIONS

Diagnosis: CXR, sputum cytology, bronchoscopy with brushings or biopsy, CT- or ultrasound-guided percutaneous biopsy, lymph node biopsy.

TNM staging: Based on tumour size, nodal involvement and metastatic spread, using CT chest, CT or MRI head and abdomen, bone scan and PET scan. Invasive methods like mediastinoscopy or video-assisted thoracoscopy may be used.

Blood: FBC, U&Es, Ca^{2+} (hypercalcaemia is common), AlkPhos (↑ bone metastases), LFT.

Pre-op: ABG, pulmonary function tests (FEV1 > 80% predicted to tolerate a pneumonectomy; lung resection is contraindicated if FEV1 < 30% predicted), V/Q scan, ECG, echocardiogram and general anaesthetic assessment.

MANAGEMENT

Multidisciplinary discussion on tumour staging and optimal treatment modality. Important considerations (surgery is not appropriate for small-cell cancer) are resectibility of the tumour (stage I and II disease, selectively IIIa) and operability (whether a patient is fit enough to undergo surgery). Frank discussion with the patient about the risks/benefits and the prognosis is vital. Only ∼14% cases are considered for surgery.

Surgery

• *Anaesthesia:* A double-lumen endotracheal tube is used to isolate the lung to be operated on from the ventilatory circuit. Central line is placed ipsilateral to the lung to be operated on. Arterial line and urinary catheter are sited. Often, a thoracic epidural catheter is placed to give good regional analgesia.

• *Procedure:* Rigid bronchoscopy is performed following induction of anaesthesia in the case of bronchial tumours. Antibiotic prophylaxis is used. Thoracotomy (usually

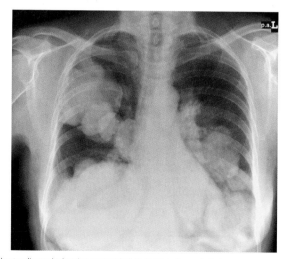

Figure 3 Chest radiograph showing cannon ball metastases (secondaries).

Lung cancer (continued)

posterolateral with the patient in a lateral decubitus position) is performed with gradual distraction of the ribs. The lung is mobilised and the position of the tumour assessed and lymph nodes inspected. Branches of the bronchial tree, pulmonary artery and vein are identified and a lobectomy performed if appropriate (~60% of resections). Bilobectomy can be performed in the right lung, with preservation of the upper or lower lobe. Sleeve resection is used to avoid pneumonectomy (involves partial resection and reconstruction of bronchi). Pneumonectomy (25% of resections) involves removal of one lung. An anterior apical drain is placed to drain air, a posterior basal drain for blood or fluid.

Non-operable: Multimodality therapy with radiotherapy and chemotherapy improves survival. Docetaxel is commonly used. Biological therapy in the form of erlotinib (inhibitor of epidermal growth factor receptor, EGFR) is a second-line chemotherapy agent.

Palliation and terminal care: Includes laser therapy to bronchial tumours, endobronchial stents, management of complications and pain control.

COMPLICATIONS

Local invasion (e.g. brachial plexus, sympathetic chain, recurrent laryngeal nerve, SVC), metastases (commonly liver, bone and brain), pleural effusion, pulmonary haemorrhage, lobar or lung collapse, paraneoplastic syndromes (particularly common in small-cell carcinomas, e.g. SIADH or ectopic ACTH production; squamous cell carcinomas are associated with hypercalcaemia of malignancy).

Surgery: Lesion unresectable at surgery (should be <5%).

Lobectomy: Air leaks are common, occasionally require re-operation.

Pneumonectomy: Considerable physiological strain due to the whole of cardiac output passing through one lung, risks of cardiac arrhythmias, failure or MI, atelectasis and pneumonia, pulmonary oedema, bronchopleural fistula, bleeding, pulmonary embolus.

PROGNOSIS

Depends on stage, but generally poor. Small-cell carcinoma is often disseminated by the time of presentation. Overall 5-year survival <5%. After resection for early stage disease, 5-year survival ~25%. Mortality of lobectomy is <2%, and mortality for pneumonectomy is 8%.

Pulmonary embolism

DEFINITION

Occlusion of pulmonary vessels, most commonly by a thrombus that has travelled to the vascular system from another site.

AETIOLOGY

Thrombus (>95% originating from DVT of the lower limbs and rarely from the right atrium in patients with atrial fibrillation). Other agents that can embolise to pulmonary vessels include amniotic fluid, air, fat, tumour and mycotic emboli from right-sided endocarditis. Groups at risk include surgical patients, and patients suffering from immobility, obesity, OCP, heart failure, malignancy.

EPIDEMIOLOGY

Relatively common, especially in hospitalised patients; occur in 10–20% of those with a confirmed proximal DVT.

HISTORY

Depends on the size and site of the pulmonary embolus.

Small: May be asymptomatic.

Moderate: Sudden onset dyspnoea, cough, haemoptysis and pleuritic chest pain.

Large (or proximal): All of the above plus severe central pleuritic chest pain, shock, collapse, acute right heart failure or sudden death.

Multiple small recurrent: Symptoms of pulmonary hypertension.

EXAMINATION

Clinical probability assessment: Various scores can predict probability to guide further investigation and management. Use local guidelines.

Well's score		Revised Geneva Score	
>4 High probability <3 Intermediate probability		>11 High probability 4–10 Intermediate probability <3 Low probability	
Clinically suspected DVT	3.0	>65 years	1
PE is most likely diagnosis	3.0	Recent surgery or fracture (1 month)	2
Recent surgery (4 weeks)	1.5	Previous DVT/PE	3
Immobilisation	1.5	Active malignancy	2
Tachycardia	1.5	Unilateral leg pain	3
History of DVT or PE	1.5	Haemoptysis	2
Haemoptysis	1.0	Heart rate >75–94/minute	3
Malignancy	1.0	Heart rate >95/minute	5
		Unilateral leg oedema and tenderness	4

Severity of pulmonary embolism can be assessed based on associated signs:
- *Small:* Often no clinical signs. Earliest sign is tachycardia or tachypnoea.
- *Moderate:* Tachypnoea, tachycardia, pleural rub, low saturation O_2 (despite oxygen supplementation).
- *Massive PE:* Shock, cyanosis, signs of right heart strain (↑ JVP, left parasternal heave, accentuated S2 heart sound).
- *Multiple recurrent PE:* Signs of pulmonary hypertension and right heart failure.

Pulmonary embolism (continued)

INVESTIGATIONS

Low probability: Use D-dimer blood test (cross-linked fibrin degradation products, sensitive but poor specificity).
High probability: Requires imaging.

Additional initial investigations:
Blood: ABG, consider thrombophilia screen.
ECG: May be normal or more commonly show a tachycardia, right axis deviation or RBBB. Classical SI, QIII or TIII pattern is relatively uncommon.
CXR: Often normal but to exclude other differential diagnoses.
Spiral CT pulmonary angiogram: First-line investigation of choice. Poor sensitivity for small emboli, but very sensitive for medium to large emboli.
Ventilation-perfusion (VQ) scan: Administration of IV ^{99}mTc macro-aggregated albumin and inhalation of krypton-81 gas. This identifies any areas of ventilation and perfusion mismatch. Not suitable if there is an abnormal CXR or coexisting lung disease due to difficulty in interpretation.
Pulmonary angiography: Gold standard, but invasive. Rarely necessary.
Doppler USS of the lower limb: To examine for venous thrombosis.
Echocardiogram: May show right heart strain.

MANAGEMENT

Primary prevention: Graduated pressure stockings (TEDs) and heparin prophylaxis in those at risk (e.g. undergoing surgery). Early mobilisation and adequate hydration post-surgery.
If haemodynamically stable: O_2, anticoagulation with heparin or LMW heparin, changing to oral warfarin therapy (INR 2–3) for a minimum of 3 months. Analgesics for pain.
If haemodynamically unstable (massive PE): Resuscitate, give oxygen, IV fluid resuscitation, thrombolysis with tPA (tissue plasminogen activator) can be considered on clinical grounds alone if cardiac arrest is imminent.
Surgical or radiological: Embolectomy (when thrombolysis is contraindicated). IVC filters (e.g. Greenfield filter) may be inserted for recurrent pulmonary emboli despite adequate anticoagulation or when anticoagulation is contraindicated.

COMPLICATIONS

Death, pulmonary infarction, pulmonary hypertension, right heart failure.

PROGNOSIS

Thirty per cent untreated mortality, 8% with treatment (due to recurrent emboli or underlying disease). Patients have ↑ risk of future thrombo-embolic disease.

Abscesses

DEFINITION

An abscess is a mass of necrotic tissue, with dead and viable neutrophils suspended in tissue breakdown products (pus), surrounded by a layer of inflammatory exudate.

AETIOLOGY

The disruption of a tissue barrier through a penetrating injury, local infection, or the migration of normal flora to sterile areas of the body becomes walled off in an attempt to limit further spread of the infection. Common bacteria include *Staphylococcus*, streptococci, enteric organisms (e.g. *Escherichia coli*), other coliforms and anaerobes (e.g. *Bacteroides* spp.). TB classically causes 'cold' abscesses. Please see **Pathology/Pathogenesis and Associations/ Risk Factors.**

ASSOCIATIONS/RISK FACTORS

- *Local*: Tissue necrosis, an underperfused space or foreign body that provides a focus for infection, e.g. a tooth or root fragment, splinters, mesh of hernia repair or embedded hair.
- *Systemic*: Diabetes, immunosuppression (although may interfere with pus formation).

EPIDEMIOLOGY

Common in all ages.

HISTORY

The patient may complain of local effects of pain, swelling, heat, redness and impaired function of the area where the abscess is present (dolor, tumour, calor, rubor and functio laesa, the Celsian features of acute inflammation) and/or systemic effects such as fever and feeling unwell.

EXAMINATION

The above features of acute inflammation are evident at the site of the abscess. If present within an organ (e.g. liver or lung, or body cavity), localising signs may be absent, the only sign being a swinging pyrexia (caused by periodic release of microbes or inflammatory mediators into the systemic circulation), which should initiate a search for an infected collection. One old adage is that if pus is somewhere and pus is nowhere, then pus is under the diaphragm (subphrenic abscess).

PATHOLOGY/PATHOGENESIS

Bacteria incite an intense acute inflammatory response with the formation of pus, a collection of cellular debris and bacteria. An abscess forms as it becomes surrounded by a fibrinous exudate and granulation tissue (macrophages and fibroblasts), with subsequent collagen deposition and walling off. Cold abscesses are collections of caseating necrosis containing mycobacterium – 'cold' because there is no associated acute inflammatory response.

INVESTIGATIONS

Bloods: FBC ($\uparrow$ neutrophils).

Imaging: Ultrasound, CT or MRI scanning or even ^{67}Ga white cell scanning may be used in the search for the site of a collection or abscess.

Aspiration: Pus is low in glucose and acidic. Culture of pus for organisms and sensitivity to antibiotics.

MANAGEMENT

Prevention: Prophylactic antibiotics (e.g. during operations), if given early during an infection. Often not effective once an abscess has formed.

General: Principles involved include drainage of pus, removal of necrotic and foreign material, antimicrobial cover and correction of the predisposing cause.

Abscesses (continued)

Surgery: Drainage of pus is carried out by incision and drainage, with debridement of the cavity and subsequent free drainage by packing of the cavity (if superficial) or by drains (if deep).

Interventional radiology: Ultrasound or CT guidance can be used to localise and aspirate the contents of an abscess.

COMPLICATIONS

Spread may result in cellulitis (in skin) or bacteraemia with systemic sepsis. If the focus of infection is not removed, a chronic abscess or discharging sinus or fistula may form. Occasionally, antibiotics may penetrate and result in the formation of a sterile collection or antibioma. If constrained by strong facial planes, slow expansion can cause pressure necrosis of surrounding tissues. Abscesses may cause destruction of normally functioning tissue (e.g. liver or nephric abscess).

PROGNOSIS

Good if adequately drained and predisposing factor removed. If left untreated, abscesses tend to 'point' to the nearest epithelial surface and may spontaneously discharge their contents. Deep abscesses may become chronic, undergoing dystrophic calcification.

Advanced trauma life support (ATLS)

INDICATIONS

Early management of trauma with emphasis on treating the greatest threat to life first.

PROCEDURE

Pre-hospital phase: Rapid assessment of the trauma patient. Treatment of hypoxaemia, shock and rapid transportation to an appropriate hospital.

Hospital phase: Primary survey is carried out by a trauma team consisting of a team leader, and usually at least a general surgeon, an orthopaedic surgeon, an anaesthetist and nursing support. The team leader should ensure a systematic approach to the primary and secondary surveys and each member of the team should have a pre-specified role.

Airway management and c-spine control: Suction and check mouth for foreign body. Check for ability to maintain own airway (conscious/unconscious patient). Chin lift/jaw thrust, oral or nasopharyngeal (not in head injury) airway as necessary, intubation or cricothyroidotomy as appropriate.

Breathing: Give oxygen, 100% via non-rebreather mask. Check for tracheal deviation and symmetrical chest expansion, bilateral breath sounds and respiratory rate. Pulse oximetry. If tension pneumothorax, needle decompression on side of pneumothorax. Check for subcutaneous emphysema. Open sucking pneumothorax requires dressing with seal on three sides and chest drain. Look for flail chest.

Circulation: Assess pulse, blood pressure, pulse pressure, capillary return, combined with intravenous access (two large-bore peripheral cannulae) and blood sampling for FBC, U&E, G&S ± crossmatch blood. Assessment of shock/haemodynamic instability, control of external haemorrhage, assessment for internal bleeding: consider major body cavities, abdomen, pelvis for signs of pelvic fractures, chest for haemothorax. Fluid resuscitation (crystalloid/colloid/blood); however, if intracavity bleeding is not yet controlled, 'permissive hypotension' of systolic BP may be appropriate (not in severe head injury where cerebral perfusion pressure should be optimized). FAST (focused abdominal sonogram for trauma) scan or CT if stable.

Disability: Assessment of neurologic injury grossly using an AVPU (Alert, Voice elicits response, Pain elicits response, Unresponsive) score or the Glasgow Coma Score (GCS). Check blood glucose.

Exposure: Check for other injuries, completely undress patient, prevent hypothermia, logroll patient, assessing for posterior or spinal injuries. Avoid and treat hypothermia: warming blankets, warm IV fluids, etc.

Frequent reassessment is key. Any deterioration requires immediate re-evaluation of the ABC. When a team is performing the assessment and resuscitation, much of the ABC may be carried out in parallel.

Secondary survey: Does not begin until the primary survey has completed and resuscitation is underway. Head-to-toe evaluation. AMPLE history (Allergies, Medications, Past illness/Pregnancy, Last meal, Events relating to the injury). Frequent reassessment vital! Full neurological examination. Radiology, and other indicated tests, e.g. FAST scan, ABG, radiographic imaging of any fractures. Urinary catheter/gastric tube. Further definitive management is dependent on injuries. Transfer to tertiary trauma or neurosurgery centre is sometimes necessary.

INVESTIGATIONS

Blood: FBC, U&E, LFTs, clotting, blood group and crossmatch as appropriate.

Urinalysis: Urine dipstick for haematuria, β-HCG if risk of pregnancy.

Imaging: Cervical spine, chest and pelvic radiographs as part of primary survey. Penetrating abdominal injury may be investigated with erect chest X-ray.

FAST scanning: Taking over as a non invasive rapid assessment for haemoperitoneum in trauma.

Advanced trauma life support (ATLS) (continued)

CT scanning: As appropriate in the stable patient. Suspicion of intra-abdominal bleed (e.g. hypotension, distended abdomen) mandates immediate laparotomy.

Radiographs: If fractured bone is suspected.

MORTALITY

Trimodal distribution of death.

- Early (within minutes) caused by large-vessel/brain/spinal cord injury.
- Second peak (within hours) due to haemorrhage, the *golden hour* refers to the period in which there is the highest likelihood that prompt medical treatment will prevent death.
- Third peak (within days to weeks) due to sepsis.

Appendicitis

DEFINITION

Acute inflammation and infection of the vermiform appendix.

AETIOLOGY

Initiated by luminal obstruction by a faecolith (inspissated faeces), lymphoid hyperplasia or oedema. Rarer causes of luminal obstruction include helminths and caecal carcinoma.

EPIDEMIOLOGY

Any age, peak incidence in the second and third decades, one of the most common emergency surgical diagnoses with a 7% lifetime risk in the UK.

HISTORY

Classic presentation (<50% of cases): Abdominal pain (usually <72 hours), initially diffuse, periumbilical and colicky (visceral pain lasting a few hours). The pain becomes sharp and localised to the RIF (somatic pain as parietal peritoneum involved). Anorexia (the most constant symptom) and nausea are common. Vomiting may occur.

Alternative presentations: Pain in the right flank (retrocaecal appendix), the right upper quadrant (long appendix) or lower abdomen (pelvic appendix). May be associated with urinary frequency or loose stools due to bladder or bowel irritation by the inflamed appendix.

EXAMINATION

Mild pyrexia, facial flush, tachycardia.

Abdominal pain often maximal at McBurney's point (2/3 along a line from the umbilicus to the anterior superior iliac spine) with rebound tenderness (demonstrable on percussion) and guarding.

Rovsing's sign: pain in the right iliac fossa elicited by pressure over the left iliac fossa.

PATHOLOGY/PATHOGENESIS

Luminal obstruction results in proliferation of bowel flora and inflammation that extends transmurally. Swelling results in obstruction and thrombosis of end arteries and the appendix becomes gangrenous and necrotic. The inflammation may become localised by omentum or bowel loops to form an appendix mass or abscess, or perforation may occur with peritonitis if not treated. Occasionally, a carcinoid tumour is found on histology; if this is >1–2 cm, a right hemicolectomy is indicated.

INVESTIGATIONS

Appendicitis is often a clinical diagnosis.

Blood: ↑ WCC and CRP, LFTs, amylase (to look for biliary pathology, pancreatitis), U&Es.

Urine: For microscopy, culture and sensitivity, pregnancy test in women of childbearing age.

Imaging: Ultrasound (often difficult to visualise appendix, useful in experienced hands, can detect other pathology, e.g. ovarian cysts). CT has 94% sensitivity and 95% specificity, especially useful if other pathology a concern, e.g. diverticulitis, but involves significant radiation exposure.

Diagnostic laparoscopy: Allows accurate diagnosis and treatment.

MANAGEMENT

General: IV fluids, broad-spectrum antibiotics pre- and perioperatively if significant signs of sepsis. If symptoms or signs are equivocal, observation with frequent re-examination.

Surgery: Appendicectomy, either open or laparoscopic (see Procedures).

Post-op: Antibiotics may be continued especially in cases of gangrenous or perforated appendix.

Appendiceal abscess: Drainage is performed either percutaneously, e.g. ultrasound or CT guided, or intraoperatively (with appendicectomy if safe). Management of an appendiceal mass may be non-operative with antibiotics, parenteral fluids and frequent reassessment,

Appendicitis (continued)

with operation if clinical deterioration. Interval appendicectomy is sometimes performed weeks later (Ochsner–Sherren approach). If this is not performed in adults, barium enema or colonoscopy should be done to exclude a carcinoma of the right colon.

COMPLICATIONS

Inflammatory mass, appendix abscess, perforation and peritonitis, rarely portal pyaemia.
Post-op: Wound infection, abscess, ileus, rarely a faecal fistula from the appendix stump.

PROGNOSIS

Appendicectomy is curative. If untreated, it can be life threatening. Diagnosis can be difficult in the very young, in the elderly and in pregnancy; morbidity and mortality in these groups are higher.

Gastrointestinal perforation

DEFINITION
Perforation of the wall of the GI tract with spillage of bowel contents.

AETIOLOGY
Gastroduodenal: Most common: perforated duodenal or gastric ulcer, more rarely gastric
carcinoma (1–2%).

Large bowel: Most common: diverticulitis and colorectal carcinoma (80%), a perforated
appendix is a common complication of appendicitis. Others: volvulus, ulcerative colitis
(toxic megacolon), trauma, radiation enteritis, post-operative anastomotic leaks or as a
complication of colonoscopy.

Small bowel (rare): Trauma, infection (typhoid, TB), Crohn's disease, lymphoma, vasculitis,
radiaton enteritis.

Oesophagus: Boerhaave's syndrome (see Oesophageal Perforation). Iatrogenic perforation
rarely occurs during OGD, more commonly during dilatation of strictures.

EPIDEMIOLOGY
Incidence depends on cause. Presentation with abdominal pain due to bowel perforation is,
however, a relatively common and potentially life-threatening emergency.

HISTORY
Depends on the cause. In general, abdominal pain, often sudden onset, associated with
nausea and vomiting.

EXAMINATION
The patient is unwell with signs of localised or generalised peritonitis with abdominal rigidity
and guarding, reduced or absent bowel sounds. Loss of liver dullness occurs due to overlying
gas. Signs of shock, pyrexia, pallor and dehydration.

INVESTIGATIONS
Blood: FBC, U&Es, LFT, amylase (levels may be raised in perforation) ABGs and clotting.

Erect CXR: May show gas under diaphragm (see Fig. 4) (70% of cases in perforated peptic
ulcer).

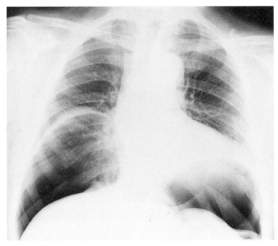

Figure 4 Erect chest radiograph showing gas under diaphragm suggestive of bowel perforation.

Gastrointestinal perforation (continued)

AXR: Can show abnormal gas shadows in tissues. *Rigler's sign* refers to gas on either side of the bowel wall; alternatively, a lateral decubitus film can demonstrate intraperitoneal gas.

CT scan: Very sensitive for free intraperitoneal gas, may also diagnose underlying pathology.

MANAGEMENT

Resuscitation: Intravenous rehydration and correction of electrolyte abnormalities, broad spectrum IV antibiotics, analgesia, urinary catheter and central line as required.

Conservative: Reserved for those with limited signs, minimal contamination or high anaesthetic risk. Treatment of gastroduodenal perforations includes bowel rest, high-dose PPIs, IV fluids and antibiotics, NG tube, monitoring.

Surgical: *Gastroduodenal*: Laparoscopy or laparotomy and peritoneal lavage: The perforation is closed and an omental patch placed. Gastric ulcers should be biopsied to examine for carcinoma. Closure is more difficult than duodenal ulcers and Billroth I partial gastrectomy with gastroduodenal anastomosis can be performed. Post-operative *Helicobacter pylori* eradication if positive.

Large bowel: Laparoscopy or laparotomy: identification of the site of perforation and peritoneal lavage. Resection of the involved colon, usually as part of a Hartmann's procedure, with formation of an end colostomy and closure of the distal stump or exteriorisation as a mucous fistula. Alternatively, resection and primary anastomosis with defunctioning ileostomy. Perforation of the right colon may allow resection and a primary anastomosis. In toxic megacolon of ulcerative colitis, a subtotal colectomy is performed with a terminal ileostomy and preservation of the rectal stump (allows future reconstruction of ileoanal pouch).

COMPLICATIONS

Sepsis, peritonitis, fistula formation, death.

PROGNOSIS

Gastroduodenal: Higher morbidity and mortality in perforated gastric ulcers than duodenal; perforated gastric carcinomas have a very poor prognosis.

Large bowel: Better prognosis with limited or local contamination. Faecal peritonitis is associated of a mortality of >50%.

Gastrointestinal stromal tumours

DEFINITION

Gastrointestinal mesenchymal tumours that may be derived from interstitial cells of Cajal, pacemaker cells associated with Auerbach's plexus that coordinate peristalsis. Exhibit a spectrum of malignant potential from very low risk to frankly malignant.

AETIOLOGY

Characterised by mutations in KIT (75–80%, CD117) or PDGFR-α (platelet-derived growth factor receptor alpha, 5–10%) resulting in a constituently activated receptor tyrosine kinase signalling pathways and cellular proliferation.

ASSOCIATIONS/RISK FACTORS

Carney's triad*, neurofibromatosis type I and familial GIST syndrome.

EPIDEMIOLOGY

Annual incidence 11–15 per million, prevalence 129 per million. Male = female, wide age distribution but 75% > 50 years (median 58 years).

HISTORY

May be asymptomatic/incidental finding at endoscopy/imaging/laparotomy. Other presentations include GI bleeding (70%), abdominal pain/bloating (57%), bowel obstruction (30%), satiety/weight loss (22%), palpable mass (13%) and more rarely, rupture.

EXAMINATION

Findings depend on site, size and complications. Can arise anywhere in the GI tract, most frequently stomach (50%), small bowel (25%), colon/rectum (10%), mesentery, omentum and retroperitoneum (10%), oesophagus (5%).

INVESTIGATIONS

Endoscopy: May reveal submucosal mass, biopsy often negative unless 'inkwell' biopsies performed. Endoscopic ultrasound: classically hypoechoic mass contiguous with the muscularis mucosa or propria. Perioperative or percutaneous biopsy is not generally recommended because of the risk of tumour rupture and spread.

Imaging: CT abdomen and ^{18}FDG PET scanning. For localising the tumour.

Immunohistochemistry: Positive for KIT (95%), CD34 (60–70%).

MANAGEMENT

Surgical resection: Treatment of choice for non-metastatic GISTs. Complete excision offers a good chance at cure and should be attempted if possible. Routine lymphadenectomy is not recommended. Laparoscopic excision can be used for small-intermediate tumours. Clinical trials of neoadjuvent and adjuvant imatinib are in progress.

Advanced disease: Imatinib binds competitively to the ATP binding site and inhibits the receptor tyrosine kinases *KIT, PDGFRA* and *BCR-ABL* and is used to treat advanced/metastatic GISTs. Disease control in up to 85% of patients with median survival >36 months. With disease progression, dose escalation or consideration of surgical resection or radiofrequency ablation of liver metastases is possible. Sunitinib is used in advanced cases that fail imatinib treatment.

COMPLICATIONS

During surgery, care should be taken to avoid tumour rupture as the risk of seeding. Modes of spread are local and haematogenous. Liver or transperitoneal metastases occur, lung/bone metastases in advanced cases; lymph node metastases are rare.

Carney's syndrome/triad: association of gastric GIST, paraganglioma and pulmonary chondroma.

Gastrointestinal stromal tumours (continued)

PROGNOSIS

Almost all GISTs have malignant potential. Prognostic factors are site, e.g. gastric more favourable outcome than small bowel, size (>5–10 cm, greater malignant potential), mitotic activity (>5 mitoses per 50 HPFs) and completeness of resection.

Hernia, femoral

DEFINITION
The abnormal protrusion of a peritoneal sac, often with abdominal contents, through the femoral canal.

AETIOLOGY
The predisposing factor is the anatomy of the femoral canal with distinct unyielding boundaries of: anteriorly the inguinal ligament, medially the lacunar ligament, posteriorly the pectineal (Cooper's) ligament and pubic bone, and laterally the femoral vein. The canal only usually consists of loose connective tissue and lymph node (Cloquet's node).

ASSOCIATIONS/RISK FACTORS
Women have a wider angle between the inguinal ligament and pectineal part of the pubic bone, hence a wider femoral canal. Raised intra-abdominal pressure predisposes to hernia formation (heavy lifting, cough or straining e.g. due to constipation or prostatism).

EPIDEMIOLOGY
Twenty-five times less common than inguinal hernias, female : male 4 : 1.

HISTORY
Present with a lump or bulge in the groin, may be uncomfortable. As femoral hernias are often small and have a tight neck, they often go unnoticed until they become strangulated or obstructed, and present as an emergency (up to 80%) with symptoms of pain, abdominal distention, nausea and vomiting.

EXAMINATION
Careful inspection will show a swelling in the groin below and lateral to the pubic tubercle (although if large, may expand up and over the inguinal ligament). There is absence of a cough impulse over the inguinal ring. If incarcerated or strangulated, the hernia may be very tender. If obstructed, abdominal distension with tinkling bowel sounds.
Differentials include inguinal hernia, lymphadenopathy, hydrocoele or lipoma of the spermatic cord (in men), groin or psoas abscess, saphaena varix or femoral aneurysm.

INVESTIGATIONS
Blood: FBC, U&Es, clotting, G&S, ABG (for metabolic acidosis in bowel ischaemia).
Imaging: *AXR*: may show bowel obstruction, USS if a different diagnosis is suspected, but should not delay surgery if an incarcerated hernia is suspected. May be an incidental finding, e.g. CT scan. Herniogram can be performed in elective cases where suspected.

MANAGEMENT
Emergency: Resuscitation with rehydration and correction of electrolyte imbalances, placement of an NG tube if vomiting, antibiotics if signs of sepsis and surgical repair as definitive treatment.
Surgery: Principles involve dissection of the sac, observing and reducing the contents, excising the sac and repairing the defect, usually by approximation of the inguinal and pectineal ligaments using non-absorbable sutures (Cooper's ligament repair). An alternative is a tension-free placement of a plug of mesh within the femoral canal. Laparoscopic mesh repair by TAPP or TEP approaches can be performed. For open surgery, there are three main approaches:
1. *Low (Lockwood)* transverse incision over the hernia (elective surgery).
2. *Transinguinal (Lotheissen)* incision above and parallel to the inguinal ligament, through the external oblique, inguinal canal and transversalis fascia (may have a higher recurrence rate).

Hernia, femoral (continued)

3. *High (McEvedy)* approach using an oblique, paramedian or unilateral Pfannenstiel incision, opening the rectus sheath, retracting the rectus medially and dividing the transversalis fascia to expose the femoral canal. This is used if strangulation is suspected. The sac is opened and contents inspected. If viable, they are reduced or if nonviable bowel is present, this is resected (may necessitate a lower midline incision if a high approach is not used).

COMPLICATIONS

Femoral hernias commonly strangulate, resulting in bowel obstruction, ischaemia and gangrene, which may necessitate surgical resection.

Surgery: Bleeding (if the lacunar ligament is incised to widen canal, an aberrant obturator artery may be injured); the risk of narrowing the femoral vein during repair can result in venous thrombosis, infection and seroma.

PROGNOSIS

Outcome is generally good with prompt and appropriate surgery, recurrence after repair is uncommon (<3%).

Hernia, inguinal

DEFINITION
The abnormal protrusion of a peritoneal sac through a weakness in the inguinal region. Indirect (60%), direct (35%) and a combination 'pantaloon' hernia (5%). Direct hernias emerge through Hesselbach's triangle (medially the lateral border of the rectus, laterally the inferior epigastric vessels and inferiorly the inguinal ligament). Hernias can be described as reducible, irreducible (incarcerated) or strangulated.

Direct: Protrusion of the hernial sac occurring directly through the transversalis fascia and posterior wall of the inguinal canal, medial to the inferior epigastric vessels.

Indirect: Protrusion of the hernial sac, through a deep inguinal ring with coverings of the spermatic cord, following the path of the inguinal canal.

AETIOLOGY
Congenital: Abdominal contents enter the inguinal canal through a persistent processus vaginalis.

Acquired: ↑ Intra-abdominal pressure together with muscle and transversalis fascia weakness. Please see **Associations/Risk Factors**.

ASSOCIATIONS/RISK FACTORS
Male, prematurity, age, raised intra-abdominal pressure, e.g. chronic cough, constipation, bladder outflow obstruction.

EPIDEMIOLOGY
Common. Congenital indirect inguinal hernias in 4% of male births. In adults peak age is 55–85 years. Men : women is 9 : 1. Ten elective repairs per 10,000 population carried out in the UK each year.

HISTORY
Asymptomatic, or the patient often notices a lump or swelling in the groin. May present due to discomfort or pain, irreducibility, ↑ in size or symptoms of complications.

EXAMINATION
Groin lump that may extend to the scrotum. Distinguished from femoral hernias by emerging above and medial to the pubic tubercle.

Examine the patient standing; the hernia is associated with a cough impulse. Indirect hernias may be controlled by pressure over the deep inguinal ring. Auscultation may reveal bowel sounds from within the hernia.

The hernia may be irreducible if incarcerated, very tender if strangulated, and may be associated with signs of complications, e.g. bowel obstruction and systemic upset, pyrexia and tachycardia.

INVESTIGATIONS
If acute with painful irreducible hernia: *Blood*: FBC, U&Es, CRP clotting and G&S if operative intervention likely. ABGs may be useful for indicating the presence of bowel ischaemia within the hernia (metabolic acidosis, ↑ lactate).

Imaging: Erect CXR and AXR in emergency cases. USS or herniogram can diagnose hernias and exclude other causes of groin lumps.

MANAGEMENT
Conservative: Patients considered unfit or unwilling to undergo surgery may be managed with an inguinal truss, a kind of belt that keeps the reduced hernia from protruding.

Surgical: Elective repair for uncomplicated hernias. Can be carried out under local, epidural, spinal or general anaesthesia. There are several types of surgical repair.

Hernia, inguinal (continued)

Mesh (Lichtenstein) repair: Oblique incision above the inguinal ligament, with opening of the external oblique aponeurosis and the spermatic cord gently freed. An indirect sac is dissected from the cord and opened (herniotomy), and the contents reduced. The sac is excised and the defect repaired, using a mesh to reinforce the defect in transversalis fascia. This is the most common procedure. Other open techniques include the Shouldice repair, which uses non-absorbable sutures to reinforce the defect, and the Stoppa repair.

Laparoscopic mesh repair: Now common, with totally extraperitoneal (TEP) and transabdominal pre-peritoneal (TAPP) approaches used. In general, laparoscopic repair results in earlier recovery and return to normal activities. The technique of choice for bilateral and recurrent hernias.

Emergency: Necessary in obstructed or strangulated hernia. Laparotomy with bowel resection may be indicated if gangrenous bowel is present within the hernia. Insertion of mesh may not be suitable in this case.

Paediatric: Indirect hernias through a patent processus vaginalis (PPV) are treated by herniotomy. The contents are reduced and the PPV is ligated, i.e. not a mesh repair.

COMPLICATIONS

Incarceration, strangulation, bowel obstruction, Maydl's hernia (strangulated W-shaped small-bowel loop), Richter's hernia (strangulation of only part of the bowel wall circumference), Amyand's hernia (acute appendicitis in a right inguinal hernia).

From surgery: Pain, wound infection, haematoma, penile or scrotal oedema, nerve damage or neuroma formation, osteitis pubis, mesh infection, testicular ischaemia, recurrence.

PROGNOSIS

Tend to slowly enlarge if left alone. Annual risk of strangulation 0.3–3%. Surgical mesh repair usually has a good outcome with recurrence in <1% of cases in mesh repairs.

Hernias, miscellaneous

DEFINITION

Classification: Hernias can be described as reducible, irreducible (incarcerated) or strangulated if there is compromise to the vascular supply of the hernia contents, e.g. omentum, bowel or abdominal organ.

Hernia Type	Description
Amyand's	When the appendix is incarcerated in an inguinal hernia
Bockdalek's	Congenital posterolateral (most often left-sided) diaphragmatic hernia
Epigastric	Herniation in the midline, through the linea alba, between the umbilicus and xiphisternum
Gluteal	Hernia through the greater sciatic foramen
Incisional	Hernia that occurs at the site of a previous surgical incision
Internal	Hernias within a body cavity, e.g. abdominal through a mesenteric defect, paraduodenal fossa, foramen of Winslow or Peterson's space following Roux-en-Y gastric bypass
Littre's	An inguinal hernia in which the sac contains a Meckel's diverticum
Lumbar	Superior (Grynfeltt–Lesshaft) or inferior (Petit) hernias
Maydl's	Hernia-en-W, i.e. contains a loop of bowel in a W formation
Morgagni	Rare congenital diaphragmatic hernia adjacent to the xiphoid process
Obturator	Herniation through the obturator foramen, producing a bulge lying below the scrotum or labial folds
Pantaloon	Simultaneous direct and indirect inguinal hernia
Parastomal	Herniation at the site of stomal orifice
Richter's	Hernias where only part of the bowel wall is trapped within the hernial sac
Sciatic	Hernia through the lesser sciatic foramen
Sliding	Where the organ, e.g. bladder or colon, forms part of the hernial sac
Spigelian	Herniation at the lateral border of rectus abdominus, at the level of the arcuate line
Umbilical and paraumbilical	Herniation through or around the umbilicus. Umbilical hernias occur in babies/children, and paraumbilical hernias in adults

AETIOLOGY

Congenital or acquired weakness in the abdominal wall and/or ↑ intra-abdominal pressure (e.g. coughing and straining) allows formation of the hernial sac.

EPIDEMIOLOGY

Incisional, epigastric, paraumbilical and parastomal hernias are relatively common. Other types are less common.

HISTORY

May be asymptomatic or notice a swelling that is painful or increasing in size.
Strangulated hernias: Tender, red and swollen hernia.
Obstruction: Initially colicky abdominal pain, nausea, vomiting and constipation.

EXAMINATION

Swelling that ↑ in size with coughing or abdominal straining.

Hernias, miscellaneous (continued)

Often non-tender and soft, but may become tender and irreducible if incarcerated or strangulated. Assess for bowel sounds or signs of obstruction in acute presentation.

INVESTIGATIONS

May be diagnosed on clinical examination, or if there is any doubt about the nature of a swelling, on imaging, e.g. USS, CT scan.

In the scenario of an acute abdomen:

Imaging: AXR, for obstruction.

Blood: FBC, U&Es, clotting, G&S, ABGs (metabolic acidosis if vascular compromise to hernia contents).

MANAGEMENT

Conservative: Asymptomatic hernias with a large neck may require no treatment.

Surgical: Elective correction is indicated for umbilical hernias persisting past 2 years of age, and symptomatic, narrow-necked or irreducible hernias. Can be performed by open or minimal access techniques. The anatomy is defined, contents inspected and reduced; the sac is excised and the defect repaired. It can be reinforced with a mesh. Emergency surgery is indicated in strangulated cases and bowel resection may be required.

COMPLICATIONS

Bowel obstruction and strangulation of hernia contents.

PROGNOSIS

Majority of umbilical hernias regress by 2 years of age. Other hernias usually do not regress and may progressively enlarge.

Hyperhidrosis

DEFINITION
A disorder of excessive sweating by eccrine glands beyond physiological requirements. Types are: primary focal, secondary generalised and localised.

AETIOLOGY
Primary focal: Stems from neurogenic sympathetic overactivity on eccrine sweat glands.

Secondary generalised: Secondary generalised hyperhidrosis can have many underlying causes, e.g. diabetes, thyrotoxicosis, hypoglycaemia, gout, pheochromocytoma, menopause, infections, e.g. TB, medication (propanolol, physostigmine, pilocarpine, tricyclic antidepressants, venlafaxine), alcoholism and malignancy.

Localised: Gustatory stimuli (Frey's syndrome), eccrine naevus, eccrine angiomatous hamartoma, Riley–Day syndrome (familial dysautonomia).

EPIDEMIOLOGY
Incidence estimated 0.6–2.8%, palmoplantar hyperhidrosis is 20× more common in Japanese ethnicity.

HISTORY
Moist hands and feet and/or axillae. Can cause social embarrassment, sometimes occupational difficulties. Patients may complain of need to frequently change clothes. Primary focal hyperhidrosis usually begins during puberty. Hyperhidrosis starting in later life should prompt search for secondary causes.

EXAMINATION
Visible sweating, may be associated with dermatitis or tinea.

Minor's iodine–starch test: Starch is brushed onto skin previously painted with 2% iodine, the light brown iodine colour turns dark purple as an iodine–starch complex forms in sweat.

INVESTIGATIONS
Only relevant for generalised hyperhidrosis.
Blood: TFTs, glucose, urate, LH/FSH, urinary catecholamines.
Imaging: As appropriate, e.g. CXR, CT or MRI scanning.

MANAGEMENT
Primary focal: First-line topical treatments, e.g. aluminium chloride, glycopyrrolate. Ionophoresis: passes a direct current across the skin, involves daily treatment of palm or sole for 30 minutes (mechanism of action unclear). Intradermal botulinum toxin injection (less pain if reconstituted in lignocaine) – effective and lasts 4–12 months. Systemic agents: anticholinergics, e.g. oxybutynin, have unappealing side-effects, dry mouth and eyes, etc.

Surgery: Thorascopic sympathectomy involves blockage of sympathetic ganglia by segmental resection, transection, cauterization or clipping of the sympathetic chain (T2/3 palmar hyperhidrosis, T3/4/5 axillary hyperhidrosis, T1 facial hyperhidrosis). Immediately effective (successful ∼95–98%).

Other techniques in axilla: Axillary skin disconnection/excision (risk of scarring, skin necrosis) or subcutaneous liposuction with dermal curettage to remove eccrine sweat glands.

COMPLICATIONS
Physical, psychological, social and occupational morbidity, skin irritation.
Of thorascopic sympathectomy: Recurrence, compensatory sweating (up to 50–60%), pneumothorax, intercostal neuralgia, Horner's syndrome.

PROGNOSIS
No increased mortality but can affect quality of life. Previously difficult to control but newer treatments are effective.

Ileus and pseudo-obstruction

DEFINITION
Functional bowel obstruction in the absence or a mechanical cause due to atony and disruption of normal peristalsis.

AETIOLOGY
Post-surgical: Bowel atony following intra-abdominal surgery.
Metabolic: Hypokalaemia, hypomagnesaemia, ketoacidosis, uraemia, porphyria, liver failure.
Infection/Inflammation: Response to inflammatory process, e.g. cholecystitis.
Diffuse peritonitis: Bacterial or chemical.
Retroperitoneal pathology: Haematoma, pancreatitis.
Drugs: Opioids, antipsychotics, anticholinergics.
Neuropathic disorders: Diabetes, multiple sclerosis, Parkinson's disease, scleroderma.
Ogilvie's syndrome: Colonic pseudo-obstruction, associated with long-term debility, chronic disease, immobility and polypharmacy.

EPIDEMIOLOGY
Depending on aetiology, but a common problem in surgical patients. Acute colonic pseudo-obstruction usually affects the elderly with underlying comorbidities.

HISTORY
History relevant to cause, e.g. recent surgery. Failure to open bowels, constipation. Initially, abdominal distension without pain, but later symptoms may mimic those of true obstruction.

EXAMINATION
Abdominal distension. Bowel sounds may be reduced or absent. Tenderness, if complications, possible peritonism. There may be faecal impaction on rectal examination.

INVESTIGATIONS
As appropriate to the patient's status and aetiology. May include the following:
Blood: FBC, U&Es, Mg^{2+}, ESR and CRP.
Imaging: Erect CXR and AXR, CT scan: may show distension of bowel, faecal impaction. Caecal diameter >12 cm significantly ↑ risk of perforation. A water-soluble contrast enema helps to differentiate from a mechanical obstruction.

MANAGEMENT
Often depends on aetiology, approaches used include the following:
Supportive: Nil by mouth, NG tube if vomiting, IV fluid replacement and correction of electrolyte imbalances, especially hypokalaemia and hypomagnesaemia. Placement of a flatus tube may help decompression. Avoidance of drugs reducing gut motility and laxatives, especially osmotic compounds, e.g. lactulose.
Medical: Treatment of the underlying cause, e.g. infection. In the absence of mechanical obstruction, persistent paralytic ileus may respond to prokinetic agents such as metoclopramide, domperidone. IV neostigmine can be used in acute colonic pseudo-obstruction, with close monitoring as risk of brochospasm, bradycardia and hypotension.
Endoscopic decompression: Can be effective in colonic pseudo-obstruction (risk of perforation ~2%).
Surgical: For imminent or realised perforation, high morbidity and mortality. Decompression and stoma formation, or if complications exist, segmental or subtotal colonic resection and exteriorization or ileorectal anastamosis.

COMPLICATIONS
Bowel perforation, most commonly caecal (40% mortality), peritonitis.

PROGNOSIS
Usually responds to conservative measures. Acute colonic pseudo-obstruction has an overall mortality rate of 25–31%.

Ingrowing toenail

DEFINITION

The lateral edge of a toenail grows into the soft tissue of the nail fold, causing inflammation and infection. The formal term is onychocryptosis.

AETIOLOGY

The toenail grows into and penetrates the skin along its margin. It can trigger a foreign body reaction, with superimposed bacterial or fungal infection. Tissue repair can result in exuberant granulation tissue formation.

ASSOCIATIONS/RISK FACTORS

Poorly fitted footware (especially those with tapering front), poorly trimmed toenails, toe trauma, poor hygiene.

EPIDEMIOLOGY

Common. More common in young adults and adolescents.

HISTORY

Pain along the margins of the toenail, painful swollen toe. Enquire about diabetes.

EXAMINATION

Erythema, oedema, warmth and tenderness, most commonly on the big toe. The lateral side of the toenail is more likely to be affected than the medial side.

INVESTIGATIONS

None usually needed.

Pus swab: Culture and sensitivity if infected.

Radiograph (toe): In severe infection and in diabetics, for osteomyelitis.

MANAGEMENT

Medical: Simple analgesia for pain and podiatry treatment. If presenting early, the foot should be regularly cleaned, with careful drying. Advice on wearing clean socks and wide-fitting shoes, and importantly to cut toenails transversely. Antibiotics may be necessary if infected (after incision and drainage if pus is present), especially in diabetics.

Surgery: For severe or recurrent cases. Ring-block local anaesthesia.

Incision and drainage: If there is a local collection of pus.

Nail avulsion: The toenail is removed without interfering with the nail bed. There is around 50% chance of recurrence.

Wedge resection: The lateral part of the nail that is ingrowing together with nail bed (~25% of the nail) is removed, using phenol to destroy the nail bed. This relieves the pressure on the sides of the toe and prevents regrowth of the nail into the skin.

Zadik's procedure: Involves removal of the entire nail and destruction of the entire nail bed.

COMPLICATIONS

Secondary infection of the nail and toe (usually fungal), deformity of nail bed and surrounding toe, permanent loss of nail.

PROGNOSIS

Generally good if treated early. Recurrence occurs in up to 30%. In diabetics, there is a higher morbidity, and can lead to loss of toe (or even limb).

Intestinal ischaemia

DEFINITION
Obstruction (e.g. by embolus or thrombosis) of a mesenteric vessel leading to bowel ischaemia and necrosis.

AETIOLOGY
Embolus (60%), arterial thrombosis (25%), venous thrombosis (15%). May be a consequence of volvulus, intussusception, bowel strangulation within a hernia or surgical resection.

ASSOCIATIONS/RISK FACTORS
Atrial fibrillation, cardiac mural thrombus and endocarditis for emboli. Hypercholesterolae-mia, hypertension, DM and smoking for arterial thrombosis. Venous thrombosis is associated with portal hypertension, splenectomy, septic thrombophlebitis, cardiac failure.

EPIDEMIOLOGY
Depends on aetiology. More common in older individuals.

HISTORY
Severe acute colicky abdominal pain. May be associated with vomiting or rectal bleeding. History of chronic mesenteric artery insufficiency (e.g. gross weight loss and abdominal pain following eating). History of heart or liver disease.

EXAMINATION
Diffuse abdominal tenderness and abdominal distension. A tender palpable mass if associated with hernia. Bowel sounds may be absent. Disproportionate degree of cardiovascular collapse.

INVESTIGATIONS
Diagnosis is difficult, may be based on clinical suspicion or found on laparotomy.
Blood: ABG (lactic acidosis), FBC, U&Es, LFT, clotting, crossmatch.
AXR: May show bowel wall thickening or thumbprinting.
CT scan: May show gas in bowel wall.
Mesenteric arteriography: If stable, allows localisation, a measure of the extent and a trial of intervention.

MANAGEMENT
General: Nil by mouth, IV fluid resuscitation and correction of electrolyte imbalances, IV antibiotics.
Surgical: Emergency laparotomy and resection of infarcted bowel. Arterial supply to non-necrotic bowel may be restored by embolectomy or by using a saphenous vein bypass from the iliac artery to the superior mesenteric artery below the obstruction. A temporary defunctioning stoma is often used. Close monitoring and care is required post-op, usually on HDU or ITU. Rarely, extensive small-bowel resection has been supported by total parenteral nutrition followed at a later stage by small-bowel transplantation.
Medical: Thrombosis prophylaxis with heparin post-op. Long-term warfarinisation may be indicated.

COMPLICATIONS
Lactic acidosis, bowel perforation, peritonitis, multi-organ dysfunction.

PROGNOSIS
A serious condition that has a high mortality (50–100%).

Intestinal obstruction

DEFINITION
Obstruction of the normal movement of bowel contents. Classified according to site: small (SBO) or large bowel (LBO), partial or complete, simple or strangulated.

AETIOLOGY
- **Simple obstruction (bowel occlusion without vascular compromise):** Intestine distal to occlusion rapidly empties and collapses while bowel above the obstruction dilates with gas and fluid. With ↑ distension, the intestinal wall blood supply becomes impaired and mucosal ulceration and bowel perforation may occur.
- **Strangulated obstruction:** The blood supply to the affected segment is compromised, leading to impairment of the normal mucosal barrier with bacterial transudation into the peritoneal cavity and peritonitis, with the unrelieved bowel developing gangrene and perforating.

The cause of the obstruction is classified into the following:
- *Extramural*: Hernia, adhesions, bands, volvulus, external compression by space-occupying lesion.
- *Intramural*: Tumours, inflammatory strictures, e.g. in Crohn's disease or diverticulitis, intussusception.
- *Intraluminal*: Pedunculated tumours, foreign bodies, e.g. bezoars, gallstones; infection, e.g. worms, constipation/faecal impaction.

EPIDEMIOLOGY
Common. More common in elderly due to increasing incidence of adhesions, hernias and malignancy.

HISTORY
Severe gripping colicky pain with periods of ease, located in the central (small intestine) or lower abdomen (large intestine).
Abdominal distension.
Frequent vomiting of greenish bile-stained vomit, early in SBO or late with faeculent vomiting in distal SBO or LBO.
Absolute constipation – failure to pass either stool or flatus.

EXAMINATION
Abdominal distension with generalised tenderness.
Visible peristalsis may be seen.
↑ Bowel sounds ('tinkling' in character). Guarding and rebound suggest peritonitis has developed, and bowel sounds may be absent.
Inspect for hernias. Any abdominal scars raise possibility of adhesions.
Inspect for abdominal mass (e.g. in intussusception, carcinoma, mass in the pouch of Douglas, faecal impaction).

INVESTIGATIONS
Blood: ABG: Lactic acidosis may suggest bowel ischaemia and impending perforation. Microcytic anaemia may indicate large bowel malignancy. Urea and electrolytes for dehydration and electrolyte disturbance secondary to vomiting.
AXR: Assists diagnosis and localisation of obstruction. Central ladder pattern of dilated loops with valvulae conniventes crossing the entire width of bowel suggest SBO. If distended bowel lies more peripherally, with haustrations that do not cross the bowel width, this suggests LBO. Fluid levels may be seen.
Erect CXR: To exclude perforation.

Intestinal obstruction (continued)

Water-soluble contrast enema: In LBO, can demonstrate the site of obstruction.

Water-soluble contrast follow-through: To investigate level of obstruction.

CT scan: Allows for pre-operative diagnosis of the cause for and/or the level of obstruction and planning of management accordingly. It may reveal metastases or perforation.

MANAGEMENT

General: Resuscitation with IV fluids and electrolyte replacement, nasogastric tube placement, close monitoring of vital signs, fluid balance, urine output and clinical status. Gastrografin follow-through may be therapeutic as well as diagnostic for adhesional obstruction. The hyperosmotic contrast is thought to reduce oedema in the bowel wall and thus, relieve the obstruction. If the study suggests an alternative diagnosis, then an early operation can be planned.

Conservative measures may settle an acute obstruction; however, if not resolving or signs of complications, operative intervention should be carried out.

Surgical: Laparotomy/laparoscopy to treat cause. May involve adhesiolysis or band division or bowel resection $+/-$ stoma. Primary anastomosis in small-bowel resection or Hartmann's operation or hemicolectomy with defunctioning stoma in large bowel resection. Post-op care in an HDU or ITU setting may be required.

Endoscopic: Obstructing colonic tumours may be stented endoscopically either pre-operatively to avoid emergency surgery, or as a palliative procedure. Obstruction secondary to a sigmoid volvulus may be treated endoscopically either with a flexible sigmoidoscope or by the passage of a flatus tube.

COMPLICATIONS

Dehydration, bowel perforation, peritonitis, toxaemia, gangrene of ischaemic bowel wall.

PROGNOSIS

Variable. Dependent on the general state of patients and the prevalence of complications.

Intussusception

DEFINITION

The process of invagination of an intestinal segment, the intussusceptum, into the adjoining intestinal lumen, the intussuscipiens, potentially resulting in vascular compromise of the bowel or obstruction.

AETIOLOGY

<3 years: Many idiopathic (up to 90%), association with lymphoid hyperplasia in Peyer's patches, Meckel's diverticulum, polyp, haematoma.

Children: Recent upper respiratory tract infections, blood dyscrasias (due to submucosal haematomas), Henoch–Schönlein purpura.

Juvenile/Adult: Mass in bowel wall or lumen, e.g. polyp, tumour, Meckel's diverticulum, approximately one-third of small-bowel cases and two-thirds of large-bowel cases are due to malignancy.

EPIDEMIOLOGY

Incidence is 1–3/1000. Usually affects <3-year-olds (majority in 3- to 9-month-olds). Rare in adults.

HISTORY

In children, intermittent episodes of severe abdominal pain, often accompanied by drawing up of legs. Bloody mucus can be passed PR that is said to resemble 'red currant jelly'.

In later stages, it can resemble bowel obstruction with vomiting and distension. In adults, symptoms can be nonspecific.

EXAMINATION

Classically, 'sausage-shaped' mass in right hypochondrium.

Signs of shock: Pale, hypotensive, tachycardia.

Signs of obstruction: Abdominal distension, tinkling bowel sounds.

Signs of peritonism: Abdominal guarding, rebound, absent bowel sounds.

PATHOLOGY/PATHOGENESIS

A pathological 'lead point' causes abnormal peristalsis and telescoping of the bowel. The ileocolic junction is the commonest site, although ileo-ileal and colo-colic also occur. Bowel wall venous congestion and oedema results, with risk of infarction and perforation if not treated.

INVESTIGATIONS

AXR: May show absence of air on the right side of the bowel or features of obstruction.

Ultrasound: Intusscepted segment appears as a target-shaped mass.

Contrast/Air enema: This is the classical way of showing intussusception, with contrast at the site showing a 'coiled spring' appearance. This can be therapeutic (see Management).

Blood: FBC, U&Es, ABG (for lactic acidosis), G&S.

MANAGEMENT

Supportive: Resuscitation with IV fluid, analgesics, antibiotic cover, NG tube insertion if vomiting.

Therapeutic enema: To reduce the invaginating segment back, can be performed with barium, air or saline. Contraindicated if there is perforation, peritonitis or suspected tumour.

Surgical: Performed in case of failure to resolve with enema or if there are signs of peritonitis. The affected bowel is gently manipulated to reduce intussusception. If the involved bowel is non-viable, cannot be reduced or Meckel's diverticulum is found, resection of the involved segment is necessary. Can be performed laparoscopically.

Intussusception (continued)

COMPLICATIONS

Can lead to ischaemia, haemorrhage, obstruction, perforation.

PROGNOSIS

Spontaneous reduction can occur in up to 10% paediatric cases. Recurrence rate is 5–10%. Good with prompt treatment, could be fatal if untreated.

Leg ulcers (venous)

DEFINITION
Ulceration of the lower limb caused by venous insufficiency, responsible for 80–85% of leg ulcers.

AETIOLOGY
Venous hypertension caused by superficial or deep venous incompetence results in increased hydrostatic pressure, tissue oedema, impaired microcirculation and eventually tissue necrosis and ulceration. Theories on mechanisms include tissue 'fibrin cuff', white cell trapping and/or chronic inflammation from ischaemia-reperfusion injury.

EPIDEMIOLOGY
Approximately 1% of the population of developed countries will develop a leg ulcer, a major burden on healthcare services, ↑ with age, female>male.

HISTORY
Chronic venous insufficiency can result in heaviness, leg aching, ankle swelling, skin changes and itching and ulceration. Determine if risk factors for deep vein thrombosis or peripheral vascular disease.

EXAMINATION
The classical position of a venous ulcer is in the 'gaiter area' above the medial malleolus.
Ulceration is often shallow, with sloping edges, surrounding skin changes of lipodermatosclerosis, varicose eczema, pigmentation or atrophie blanche.
Examine for varicose veins with the patient standing.
Determine ankle–brachial pressure index (ABPI) to look for concurrent peripheral arterial disease.
Differential diagnosis includes arterial, diabetic, neuropathic, vasculitic, infective and neoplastic ulcers.

INVESTIGATIONS
Ankle–brachial pressure index (ABPI): All patients should be screened for arterial disease using ABPIs. For those with ABPI 0.5–0.8, modified compression may be possible and <0.5 should be referred/assessed for management of arterial insufficiency in the first instance.
Microbiology swab: If signs of infection, e.g. discharge, erythema, cellulitis or pyrexia.
Biopsy or cytology: If any concern about malignancy.

MANAGEMENT
Multi-component compression bandaging: Correction of venous hypertension by multi-layer compression, e.g. Charing Cross four-layer bandage of wool, crepe, elastic and cohesive bandages. Advice on leg elevation and mobility. Once healed, compression stockings prevent recurrence. Antibiotics should be reserved for infected ulcers with surrounding cellulitis. Pentoxifylline may be a beneficial adjunct. Topical applications, routine systemic antibiotics and type of dressing have not been shown to improve healing.
Surgery: Endovascular or open surgical treatment of varicose veins. The ESCHAR (Effect of Surgery and Compression on Healing and Recurrence) study showed that superficial venous surgery does not speed healing by compression but, once healed, helps prevent recurrence. Skin grafting may be appropriate in selected patients.

Leg ulcers (venous) (continued)

COMPLICATIONS

Chronic wounds, infection, recurrence, development of malignancy in long-standing ulcers (Marjolin's ulcer).

PROGNOSIS

Often a chronic problem, with variable healing rates. After healing, recurrence rates are approximately 25% at one year and 33% at 18 months.

Lipomas

DEFINITION

Lipomas are slow-growing benign tumours of adipose tissue. Lipomatosis refers to multiple contiguous lipomas that cause distortion of tissues (e.g. on buttock or, rarely, neck). Can be classified by location, e.g. subcutaneous, subfascial, subsynovial.

AETIOLOGY

Can arise in any connective tissue but are most common in subcutaneous fat. Histologically, lipomas are made up of collections of adipose cells indistinguishable from normal adipocytes divided into large lobules by thin fibrous septa.

Unknown cause, certain chromosomal aberrations have been implicated (e.g. translocation of a gene on chromosome 12). A rare presentation is multiple tender lipomas (Dercum's disease/adiposis dolorosa).

EPIDEMIOLOGY

All ages, mostly 40–60 years, rare in children. No gender preference.

HISTORY

Patient notices a lump, usually painless and slowly enlarging, unless subject to trauma when fat necrosis may cause it to swell and become tender.

EXAMINATION

Can occur anywhere where there are adipose tissue reserves, common in the subcutaneous tissue of the upper arms. Variable size, usually ovoid or spherical, often lobulated (a useful diagnosic feature). Non-tender, soft, compressible, but do not usually fluctuate or transilluminate. The overlying skin is usually normal. Local lymph nodes should not be palpable.

INVESTIGATIONS

Usually none necessary; MRI can be used for visualising deeply sited lipomas.

MANAGEMENT

Conservative: May be left alone if not causing discomfort or distorting appearance.

Surgical: If troublesome or unsightly. Can be removed under local anaesthesia: An incision is made over the lipoma to expose it; a typical feature is that the lipoma can be milked out through the incision by gentle pressure on the surrounding tissue, often with minimal dissection. Haemostasis in the resulting cavity should be ensured to avoid haematoma development. Larger lipomas or those in more complicated sites will need excision under general anaesthetic.

COMPLICATIONS

Usually associated with surgery to remove them rather than the lipoma itself.
If traumatised, may undergo fat necrosis.

PROGNOSIS

Excellent; as a general rule, lipomas do not become malignant (liposarcomas usually arise de novo, e.g. in the retroperitoneum).

Meckel's diverticulum

DEFINITION

True congenital small-bowel diverticulum on the antimesenteric border of the ileum. Follows the rule of 2s: 'occurs in 2% of the population, is 2 ft from the ileocaecal valve, is 2 in in length'.

AETIOLOGY

In an embryo, the omphalomesenteric/vitelline duct connects the developing midgut to the yolk sac. Failure of the duct to completely regress during 5th–7th week can result in a persistent diverticulum or more rarely in an omphalomesenteric fistula, sinus, fibrous band or vitelline duct cyst.

EPIDEMIOLOGY

Most common congenital anomaly of the small intestine, 2% of the population, male = female but 2–4 times more symptomatic in males; at any age, ~60% become so before the age of 10 years.

HISTORY

Most commonly asymptomatic/incidental finding. PR bleeding (most commonly in children), usually painless dark or red blood (brick red) mixed with stool and can be major and associated with shock. Abdominal pain due to diverticulitis/ulceration. Symptoms of bowel obstruction due to volvulus or intussusception. Rarely, mucoid or purulent discharge from the umbilicus.

EXAMINATION

Signs can be minimal. With bleeding there may be signs of shock. Guarding/rebound tenderness due to inflammation can mimic signs of acute appendicitis.

PATHOLOGY/PATHOGENESIS

A true diverticulum (varies from 0.5 to 50 cm) contains all layers of the bowel wall, lined by small intestinal mucosa, but commonly contains heterotopic tissue (5% of asymptomatic and 60% of symptomatic cases), often gastric or pancreatic mucosa (but rarely duodenal, jejunal or colonic). Ectopic gastric mucosa secretes acid that can cause erosion or bleeding.

INVESTIGATIONS

Bloods: If bleeding, FBC, U&E, clotting, crossmatch.

Isotope scan: ^{99m}Tc-pertechnetate is taken up by a Meckel's diverticulum if ectopic gastric mucosa is present (however, a negative scan does not exclude its presence). Pre-operative diagnosis is difficult. May be seen during barium contrast studies.

AXR, erect CXR: If signs of obstruction or perforation.

Mesenteric angiography: May be useful in cases of active bleeding; however, this may not be sensitive if bleeding is slow.

MANAGEMENT

Emergency (bleeding or obstruction): Resuscitation with correction of fluid and electrolyte abnormalities.

Surgical: Surgical resection (diverticulectomy) with or without small-bowel resection and division of bands. There is no compelling evidence for resection of incidental Meckel's diverticulum, but this can be performed laparoscopically with endostaplers.

COMPLICATIONS

Cumulative risk over lifetime ~6%: bleeding, obstruction secondary to an internal hernia around an omphalomesenteric band, inflammation (diverticulitis), intussusception or enterolith. Littre's hernia is one in which there is incarceration of a Meckel's diverticulum. Carcinoid tumours within Meckel's diverticulum have been reported.

PROGNOSIS

Usually good with appropriate management.

Nutrition

DEFINITION

Oral nutritional support: Provision of fortified foods and/or supplements.

Enteral nutrition: Delivered via the GI tract, includes oral nutritional supplements and tube feeding by oral, nasal or percutaneous routes.

Parenteral nutrition: Intravenous provision of nutrients, electrolytes and fluid.

EPIDEMIOLOGY

Approximately 40% patients are malnourished on admission.

HISTORY

Weight loss, poor appetite, symptoms of associated illness or complications.

EXAMINATION

Physical appearance, signs of cachexia. Anthropometric measurements: weight, BMI, mid-arm circumference, triceps skin-fold thickness.

PATHOLOGY/PATHOGENESIS

Glucose is initially supplied by glycogen breakdown in the liver. After 24 hours hepatic gluconeogenesis occurs (using glycerol from fatty acids, aminoacids from protein breakdown). Lipolysis releases glycerol and free fatty acids, which are metabolised by the liver to ketone bodies.

INVESTIGATIONS

Nutritional screening/assessment on admission, SGA (subjective global assessment), albumin, Ca, Mg, PO_4, Zn.

MANAGEMENT

Should be coordinated/monitored by a multi-disciplinary team consisting of a dietitian, SALT and medical team.

Indications:

- *Oral nutritional support*: Those at risk or malnourished (defined by a BMI <18.5 kg/m^2, unintentional weight loss >10% in the previous 3–6 months or a BMI <20 and unintentional weight loss >5% in the previous 3–6 months).
- *Enteral*: Malnutrition, dysphagia, upper GI obstruction (stricture, tumour), sedation (in ICU). Nasojejunal: pancreatitis (decreases infective complications and improves mortality in severe pancreatitis), poor gastric motility, gastric outflow obstruction, patients at risk of aspiration.
- *Parenteral*: When gastrointestinal tract is not functioning or available, e.g. short bowel syndrome, high fistula, prolonged ileus/obstruction.

Contraindications:

- *Enteral*: Bowel obstruction, absent peristalsis, terminal disease (unless patient wishes).
- *Parenteral*: Caution in renal and liver failure, egg/soya allergy.

Feeds: Enteric formulae can be nutritionally complete or incomplete (supplement only). Standard formulae contain macro- and micronutrients, whole protein, lipid (long-chain triglycerides) with or without fibre. *Others*: disease-specific formulae, immune-modulating, low- or high-energy, high-protein, whole-protein, peptide-based, free amino acid (elemental), high-lipid, and highly mono-unsaturated fatty acid formulae.

Routes of enteral feeding: Tube feeding via nasogastric, orogastric, nasojejunal, percutaneous endoscopic gastrostomy (PEG), PEG with jejunal extension, radiologically inserted gastrostomy (RIG), or surgical jejunostomy.

Parenteral feeding (TPN): Usually delivered by central venous access, but can be formulated for peripheral routes. Monitoring while on TPN:

- *Daily*: U&E, LFT, PO_4, Ca^{2+}, Mg^{2+}, glucose, Alb, CRP, Hb, WCC (after initial 5 days, do above 3× a week unless problems).

Nutrition (continued)

- *Weekly*: Triglycerides, iron studies.
- *Monthly*: Selenium, copper, zinc, manganese, vitamin A, vitamin E.

COMPLICATIONS

Malnutrition: Impaired wound healing, immune dysfunction, muscle weakness, ↑ susceptibility to infection, pressure sores, ↑ hospital stay, ↑ readmission rates, ↑ mortality.

Enteral feeding: *Biochemical*: Refeeding syndrome (potentially fatal metabolic shift when patients with depleted body stores of minerals such as K, Mg and PO_4 have a carbohydrate source administered, characterised by hypophosphataemia, hypokalaemia and hypomagnesaemia), fatty liver, impaired renal function.

Mechanical: Diarrhoea, vomiting, nausea, abdominal pain.

Parenteral feeding: *Line related*: Sepsis, thrombosis.

Feed related: Metabolic acidosis, deranged LFTs & fatty liver, hyperglycaemia, bacterial translocation, renal failure, acute cholecystitis (bile stasis), refeeding syndrome.

PROGNOSIS

Malnourished patients have 2–3× more complications than nourished counterparts.

Pain management

INDICATION

Perioperatively, pain can arise from the surgical procedure, complications, drains/invasive investigations or pre-existing disease. Pain is associated with physical, psychological and emotional distress. Appropriate treatment leads to faster recovery and return to normal activity, shorter hospital stay and improved patient satisfaction.

INVESTIGATIONS

Pre-op: *Patient characteristics to consider*: age, diagnosis, pre-morbid pain status, opioid exposure, comorbidities – renal and hepatic impairment, anxiety disorder, cultural factors. Appropriate explanation, reassurance and discussion about options for management with patients pre-operatively will allay fears and help reduce anxiety.

Post-op: *Frequent pain assessment*: location, quality, severity, temporal pattern, constant versus intermittent, aggravating and relieving factors. Methods to quantify pain level include numeric rating scales (e.g. '1 to 10') or visual analogue scales (e.g. faces, used for children). Once analgesia is administered, it is important to evaluate the response and review/revise as needed. Always be aware that unexpected, unexplained or excessive pain may be a sign of a complication; this should be flagged and investigated in addition to pain management.

PAIN CONTROL

Pain control should be multi-modal, i.e. best treated not by a single drug or therapy but by combinations, which maximise efficacy whilst keeping side-effects low. The WHO analgesic ladder is a framework for prescription of analgesic drugs, developed originally to improve management of cancer pain.

Pharmacological analgesics: Summarised in the following tables.

Standard analgesics				
Class	**Effects**	**Mechanism**	**Side-effects**	**Administration**
Local anaesthetics	Analgesic, often given in combination with opioid in epidurals	Inhibit sodium channels and reduce transmission along pain nerve fibres.	Hypotension due to sympathetic blockade, can cause neuromuscular blockade. Toxicity: cardiac dysrhythmias, hypertension, dizziness, paraesthesias, seizures, coma	Topical (EMLA cream), local wound infiltration, nerve blocks or delivery via regional catheter, epidural
Paracetamol	Analgesic, antipyretic	Still debated, reduces prostaglandin production by COX inhibition	Risk of hepatic failure in overdose	Oral, rectal, intravenous
NSAIDs	Analgesic, antipyretic, anti-inflammatory	Inhibit cyclo-oxygenase and prostaglandin production	Bronchospasm, GI erosions, renal impairment, platelet dysfunction	Oral, rectal, IV

Pain management (continued)

Standard analgesics				
Class	Effects	Mechanism	Side-effects	Administration
Opioids	Analgesic, euphoria, sedation, cough suppression, anxiolytic	Act as agonists on mu, kappa and delta receptors	Respiratory depression, nausea and vomiting, urinary retention, constipation, pruritis, tolerance, dependence	Oral, IM, SC, IV, e.g. patient-controlled analgesia (PCA), transdermal patch

Adjuvant analgesics				
Class	Effects	Mechanism	Side-effects	Administration
Low-dose antidepres-sants (e.g. tricyclics)	Used in neuro-pathic pain	Inhibit reuptake of serotonin and noradrenaline neurotransmitters.	Anticholinergic effects: dry mouth, drowsiness, constipation, urinary retention	Oral
Anticon-vulants (e.g. gabepentin)	Used in neuro-pathic pain, phantom limb pain	Gabapentin is a GABA analogue but mechanism is unclear, thought to bind to voltage-dependent calcium channel in the CNS	Gabapentin: dizziness, drowsiness, ataxia, peripheral oedema	Oral
Muscle relaxants (e.g. diazepam)	Muscle relaxation, anxiolysis, anti-convulant	Benzodiazepines bind to GABA-A receptors to enhance the inhibitory effect of GABA	Drowsiness, suppression of REM sleep, impaired motor function, amnesia, dizziness, tolerance, physical dependence	Oral, rectal, IV, IM

Non-pharmacological pain control methods: Explanation, education, hypnosis, cold or heat application, splinting of wounds, transcutaneous electrical nerve stimulation (TENS), neurolytic blocks, acupuncture.

COMPLICATIONS

Of under-treatment: Emotional and physical suffering, sleep disturbance, delayed mobilisation and thromboembolism; respiratory complications: atelectasis, sputum retention; autonomic stimulation: hypertension, tachycardia, increased myocardial oxygen consumption and stress, impaired wound healing, tachypnea.

Psychological: Anxiety, depression, anger, hostility suffering.

Peritonitis

DEFINITION

Peritonitis is inflammation of the peritoneal lining of the abdominal cavity and can be localised or generalised; the latter can be primary or secondary.

AETIOLOGY

Localised: Common causes are appendicitis, cholecystitis, diverticulitis, salpingitis.

Primary generalised: Bacterial infection of the peritoneal cavity without obvious focus responsible. Primary pneumococcal peritonitis due to *Streptococcus penumoniae* can occur in children. In adults, often associated with cirrhosis and ascites (spontaneous bacterial peritonitis) or renal failure patients having CAPD (continuous ambulatory peritoneal dialysis).

Secondary generalised: Peritonitis spreads from a localised infective focus, usually polymicrobial (see above) or nonbacterial due to spillage of bile, blood, gastric contents, e.g. perforated peptic ulcer, pancreatic secretions (a chemical peritonitis that often becomes secondarily infected).

EPIDEMIOLOGY

Primary peritonitis is rare and usually presents in adolescent females; localised and secondary generalised peritonitis are very common.

HISTORY

A careful history should be taken with exploration of the onset, nature, course and radiation of the abdominal pain as well as exacerbating, relieving and associated factors. Parietal pain from peritonitis is usually continuous, sharp, localised and exacerbated by movement and coughing (parietal peritoneum is supplied by somatic A-δ fibres arising from spinal nerves of T7–L2).

EXAMINATION

Assess vital signs, signs of dehydration or compromised perfusion (e.g. due to hypovolaemia, sepsis or circulatory failure).

Localised: Tenderness with involuntary guarding: reflex contraction of overlying abdominal wall muscles; rebound tenderness: sudden removal of a palpating hand causes pain due to movement of the inflamed peritoneum, similarly demonstrated as percussion tenderness or pain evoked by coughing.

Generalised: The patient is usually very unwell with systemic signs of toxaemia or sepsis (e.g. fever, tachycardia); movement exacerbates pain. The abdomen is rigid with generalised guarding and rebound, and bowel sounds are reduced or more typically absent due to paralytic ileus.

INVESTIGATIONS

As indicated by history and clinical assessment.

Blood: FBC, U&Es, LFT, amylase, CRP, clotting, G&S or crossmatch, blood cultures, pregnancy test, ABG (looking for metabolic acidosis, lactate levels or respiratory failure).

Erect CXR: For pneumoperitoneum.

AXR: For bowel obstruction.

CT abdomen or laparoscopy: To diagnose the cause of the peritonitis. When inflamed, the peritoneum loses its glistening appearance and becomes erythematous with production of copious serous inflammatory exudate, rich in white blood cells, protein and inflammatory mediators. The greater omentum becomes adherent to inflamed organ, providing a barrier to spread of infection.

If ascites: Ascitic tap and cell count (diagnostic of SBP if >250 neutrophils/mm^3), Gram stain and culture.

Peritonitis (continued)

Localised: Treatment will depend on underlying cause (e.g. appendicectomy in appendicitis), IV antibiotics (e.g. cholecystitis, salpingitis and most cases of acute diverticulitis).

Generalised: The patient is at risk of death from sepsis and shock. Needs IV fluid resuscitation and correction of volume and electrolyte imbalance and IV antibiotics. Urinary catheter, NG tube and CVP line to monitor fluid balance and appropriate surgical intervention.

Urgent laparotomy/laparoscopy: To identify and treat cause, remove infected or necrotic tissue and perform copious peritoneal lavage. An exception would be acute non-necrotising pancreatitis.

Primary peritonitis: Treated with antibiotics, but this diagnosis is often not apparent until after attempted operative intervention.

Early: Septic shock, respiratory or multi-organ failure, paralytic ileus, wound infection, tertiary peritonitis (persistence of intra-abdominal infection), abscesses, portal pyaemia/hepatic abscesses.

Late: Incisional hernia, adhesions.

With appropriate treatment of the underlying cause, localised peritonitis usually resolves. Generalised peritonitis has a much higher mortality, approaching 30–50%. The concurrent development of septic shock or multi-organ dysfunction can ↑ the mortality rate to >70%. Primary peritonitis has a good prognosis with appropriate antibiotic therapy. The overall mortality rate of patients with SBP may exceed 30% if diagnosis and treatment are delayed.

Pilonidal sinus

DEFINITION
A pilonidal sinus (Latin for 'nest of hair') is an abnormal epithelium-lined tract filled with hair that opens to the skin surface, most commonly in the natal cleft.

AETIOLOGY
Proposed to be caused by shed or sheared hairs penetrating the skin and inciting an inflammatory reaction and sinus development, with intermittent negative pressure drawing in more hair and perpetuating the cycle.

EPIDEMIOLOGY
Common, annual incidence of 26 per 100,000, male > female, mean age of presentation 19 (women) and 21 years (men).
Associated with hirsute individuals, certain occupations may predispose; e.g. hairdressers may develop interdigital pilonidal sinus. Known as 'jeep bottom' due to soldiers developing the condition during World War II.

HISTORY
Painful natal cleft, especially if inflamed or superimposed infection, and the patient may complain of associated discharge or swelling. Often a recurrent problem.

EXAMINATION
Midline openings or pits are seen between the buttocks, from which hairs may protrude. If associated infection or abscess, a tender swelling develops that may be fluctuant or discharge pus or bloodstained fluid on compression. Secondary openings or pits are common.

PATHOLOGY/PATHOGENESIS
The sinus tract is lined with squamous epithelium and extends a variable distance into subcutaneous tissue, often with branching side channels. Hair shafts and foreign body giant cells are seen in associated granulation tissue. Tracking of bacteria leads eventually to inflammation and the formation of a polymicrobial abscess filled with granulation tissue, pus and hair.

INVESTIGATIONS
None needed for diagnosis. If infection raised WCC, check glucose (for diabetes).

MANAGEMENT
Acute pilonidal abscess: Usually requires incision and drainage (can be done under local anaesthesia if small) for evacuation of pus and hair. The cavity is irrigated and packed, and dressings changed regularly until there is secondary closure. Antibiotic cover post-op is usually unnecessary.

Chronic pilonidal sinus: Treatment principles involve sinus tract excision, skin healing and prevention of recurrence. Excision under general anaesthesia with exploration, laying open and removal of tracts (may be identified by staining with methylene blue). The fibrous tissue tracts attached to the sacrococcygeal bone can be divided. Wound closure by either primary closure, either midline or off midline, or left open and healing by secondary intention. Wounds closed primarily heal more quickly, but there is increased risk of recurrence. Wounds off the midline heal better and have less chance of recurrence.

- *Karydakis operation*: Asymmetric excision with a lateral closure, flattens and lateralizes the midline cleft.
- *Bascom technique*: Excision of midline pits and closure, then a lateral incision to removal of the chronic abscess cavity, leaving the lateral wound open.

Prevention by attention to hygiene in the area; depilation or shaving is important in preventing recurrence.

Pilonidal sinus (continued)

COMPLICATIONS

Pain, infection, abscess, recurrence.

PROGNOSIS

Good with appropriate management. Complicated disease can be troublesome and cause recurrent infection. Usually resolves by age of 40.

Sebaceous cysts

DEFINITION

Epithelium-lined, keratinous, debris-filled cyst arising from a blocked hair follicle. More correctly known as epidermal cyst.

AETIOLOGY

Occlusion of the pilosebaceous gland. More frequent in Gardner's syndrome.

EPIDEMIOLOGY

Extremely common, any age.

HISTORY

Non-tender slow-growing skin swelling, often multiple. May become red, hot and tender if superimposed inflammation or infection.

EXAMINATION

Smooth tethered lump in the skin with overlying punctum.
Common on hair-bearing areas of the body, especially scalp, trunk or scrotum.
May express granular creamy material with an unpleasant smell.

PATHOLOGY/PATHOGENESIS

Despite their name, these cysts are not derived from sebaceous glands. Sebaceous cysts result from the cystic proliferation of epidermal cells within the dermis. The source of this epidermis is often the infundibulum of the hair follicle.

INVESTIGATIONS

None usually required. Excision biopsy or FNA rarely necessary.

MANAGEMENT

Conservative: May be left alone if not causing the patient distress.

Surgical: Excision of cyst can be carried out under local anaesthesia. Care must be taken to ensure complete removal or the cyst is liable to recur. If an abscess develops in association, it should be drained.

Medical: If there is infection, antibiotics may be given; however, definitive treatment involves excision once acute inflammation has settled.

COMPLICATIONS

Infection, abscess formation. Recurrence if excision is incomplete. Occasionally, may ulcerate and have the appearance of a skin malignancy (Cock's peculiar tumour). A sebaceous horn may develop if the discharging contents dry out and form a horn-shaped protrusion.

PROGNOSIS

Excellent; most do not require treatment and excision is usually curative.

Systemic inflammatory response syndrome (SIRS) and sepsis

DEFINITION
SIRS: When two or more of the following are present:
- Heart rate >90/minute.
- Temperature <36 °C or >38 °C.
- Tachypnoea >20/minute or $PaCO_2 < 4.3$ kPa (32 mmHg).
- WCC < 4000 or >12,000 cells/mm^3 or >10% immature neutrophils.

Sepsis: SIRS + infection.
Severe sepsis: Sepsis + organ dysfunction, hypotension or hypoperfusion.
Septic shock: Sepsis-induced hypotension despite adequate fluid resuscitation.

AETIOLOGY
SIRS is a common inflammatory response to a wide variety of physiological insults, can be caused by infection, ischaemia, inflammation, e.g. pancreatitis, trauma, burns. Can progress to multiple organ dysfunction syndrome (MODS): altered organ function in an acutely ill patient such that haemostasis cannot be maintained without intervention.

EPIDEMIOLOGY
All ages, extremes of age and concomitant comorbidities negatively affect the outcome.

HISTORY
Depends on the aetiology whether infectious, traumatic, ischaemic or inflammatory.

EXAMINATION
Thorough systematic examination for diagnosis with attention to vital signs, urine output, mental status. Respiratory rate is a sensitive sign of severity of illness.

PATHOLOGY/PATHOGENESIS
Following an insult, local cytokines incite an inflammatory response to fight infection and promote healing. Cytokines are released into circulation to improve the local response. This acute-phase response is usually controlled by a decrease in the pro-inflammatory mediators and by the release of endogenous antagonists. If homeostasis is not restored, a cycle of uncontrolled pro-inflammatory amplification arises, with inflammation and coagulation dominant resulting in microcirculatory thrombosis, hypoperfusion, ischaemia, loss of circulatory integrity and tissue injury.

INVESTIGATIONS
Blood: FBC, U&E, LFT, amylase, cardiac enzymes. Inflammatory markers include CRP and ESR, with newer IL6, IL8, pro-calcitonin and LPS-binding protein.
ABG: Provides important information on severity of acidosis, lactate.
Cultures: Blood, sputum, urine, lines, other potentially infected sites CSF, joint fluid, ascites or pleural effusions.
Imaging studies: To locate/sample source of infection.

MANAGEMENT
Immediate stabilisation of the patient: Resuscitation according to ABC. In sepsis, prompt institution of empirical antibiotics and support organ function. Targeted and protocol-driven early 'goal-directed therapy' of fluid and inotropic support has been shown to improve the outcome from sepsis with a standardised approach formulated into the *Surviving Sepsis Campaign*. Goals include the following:
- Central venous pressure 8–12 mmHg
- Mean arterial pressure ≥65 mmHg
- Urine output ≥0.5 ml/kg/hour
- Central venous oxygen saturation ≥70%

Supportive measures: Critical care support, glycaemic control, nutrition, DVT and stress ulcer prophylaxis. Acute renal failure often develops during severe sepsis and may require renal replacement therapy. Even if renal function is normal in a septic patient, early high-volume continuous veno-venous haemofiltration may still be advocated. It is thought that this process may remove some of the pro-inflammatory or pro-coagulant cytokines that drive the septic cascade.

Activated protein C: The PROWESS study showed that recombinant-activated protein C (drotrecogin alpha) reduces mortality in severe sepsis (increased risk of bleeding).

Surgical: Acute surgical problems should be managed appropriately, e.g. drainage of abscesses, removal/debridement of infected tissue.

COMPLICATIONS

Multi-organ dysfunction; renal failure, coagulopathy, liver failure, ARDS, death.

PROGNOSIS

Mortality rates: SIRS ~7%, severe sepsis 30% and septic shock (>50%). Mortality rates increase by 15–20% for each additional organ failure.

Splenic rupture

DEFINITION
Rupture of the spleen causing risk of major intra-abdominal haemorrhage.

Severity rating (American Association for the Surgery of Trauma)
- *Grade 1*: Minor subcapsular tear (<1 cm) or haematoma (<10% of surface area)
- *Grade 2*: Nonexpanding subcapsular haematoma 10–50% of surface area, intraparenchymal haematoma <5 cm in diameter
- *Grade 3*: Subcapsular haematoma >50% of surface area, intraparenchymal haematoma >5 cm, laceration >3 cm or involving trabecular vessels, ruptured subcapsular or intraparenchymal haematoma
- *Grade 4*: Laceration involving segmental or hilar vessels with major devascularisation
- *Grade 5*: Shattered spleen, hilar vascular injury with devascularised spleen

AETIOLOGY
Most frequently due to non-penetrating trauma or rapid deceleration injury. Associated with other traumatic internal organ injury, e.g. liver, kidney, pancreas and diaphragm as well as rib fractures. Splenomegaly and its causes such as infectious mononucleosis, malaria and leukaemia ↑ the risk of rupture from even minor trauma.

EPIDEMIOLOGY
Relatively common, some degree present in up to 25% of major trauma cases.

HISTORY
History of blunt trauma. Abdominal pain that may be diffuse or localised to the left flank, and may result in referred pain to the left shoulder tip (Kehr's sign).

EXAMINATION
Abdominal tenderness, guarding and rigidity (generalised or left flank only).
Signs of shock (e.g. hypotension, tachycardia).
There may be delayed rupture by up to several days post-trauma due to the formation of a subcapsular haematoma that expands in size eventually rupturing.

INVESTIGATIONS
Blood: FBC, U&Es, LFTs, clotting and crossmatch.
Ultrasound: Focused assessment with sonography for trauma to detect for fluid in the peritoneal cavity suggestive of intra-abdominal haemorrhage.
CT scan: To identify splenic trauma as well as trauma to other organs.
CXR: May show rib fractures, diaphragmatic rupture or left pulmonary contusion.
Diagnostic peritoneal lavage: Detects free intraperitoneal blood – rarely performed due to availability of FAST and CT scanning.

MANAGEMENT
Depends on the heamodynamic state and grade of injury.
Resuscitation: Wide-bore IV access, fluids, transfusion if necessary, avoiding overinfusion (permissive hypotension may be tolerated).
- *Grade 1 and some Grade 2*: Manage conservatively with close monitoring and regular review. Consider interventional radiological techniques to embolise a bleeding point.
- *Grade 3*: Laparotomy and possible splenorrhaphy/splenectomy.
- *Grades 4 and 5*: Splenectomy.

Post-op: Immunisation against pneumococcal, meningococcal (Men C) and haemophilus organisms should be given. Antibiotic prophylaxis is also given up to the age of 15 with patients keeping a home supply of antibiotics to take at any sign of infection.

COMPLICATIONS

From injury: Haemorrhage, death.

From splenectomy: Haemorrhage, post-splenectomy sepsis, ↑ risk of encapsulated organism infections, thrombotic vascular event (splenic/splanchnic venous thrombosis), pancreatic injury, pancreatitis, subphrenic abscess, gastric distension, focal gastric necrosis.

From splenorrhaphy: Rebleeding or thrombosis of remaining spleen.

PROGNOSIS

Seventy-five per cent mortality if untreated. With treatment, mean mortality ranges from 3% to 23%.

Branchial cyst, sinus and fistula

DEFINITION
Neck swelling or discharge that arises from incomplete obliteration of pharyngeal clefts and pouches during embryonic development.

AETIOLOGY
Ninety-five per cent arise from congenital remnants of the second pharyngeal pouch or branchial cleft, although the precise embryological origin is disputed (possibly incomplete involution or ectopic tissue).

EPIDEMIOLOGY
Uncommon. Branchial cysts are the most common, presenting most often in the third decade, with considerable variation. Fistulae and sinuses usually present in children.

HISTORY
The patient complains of a lateral neck swelling that may vary in size over time; it is usually painless unless inflammation and infection develop, then becomes painful and red. A sinus or fistula presents with a neck dimple that discharges mucus or mucopurulent fluid.

EXAMINATION
If this is a cyst, a lump is present just deep to sternocleidomastoid at the junction of its upper and lower two-thirds.
On palpation the swelling is usually ovoid, smooth and firm, may be relatively soft in early stages, fluctuant and may transilluminate. Two per cent are bilateral.
The external opening of a branchial sinus or fistula is at the junction of the middle and lower one-third of the anterior edge of sternocleidomastoid.

PATHOLOGY/PATHOGENESIS
Grooves in the neck, known as branchial clefts, with the intervening branchial arches appear in the 5th week of foetal development. The first cleft persists as the external auditory meatus, but the remainder normally disappear. If remnants of the second cleft remain, a cyst, sinus or fistula may develop. The cysts are lined by squamous or respiratory epithelium and contain collections of turbid fluid consisting of epithelial debris and cholesterol crystals, some contain lymphoid tissue.
A branchial fistula passes between the internal and external carotid arteries, superior to the hypoglossal nerve and inferior to the glossopharyngeal nerve terminating in the posterior part of the tonsillar fossa in the oropharynx.

INVESTIGATIONS
Imaging: Ultrasound, CT or MRI scanning can be used to visualise the cyst.
FNA: Used to distinguish from cervical lymph node metastases in older individuals (e.g. thyroid cancer and mucoepidermoid carcinomas of salivary glands that may have a significant cystic component).

MANAGEMENT
Surgery: Treatment is surgical excision of the cyst and any associated sinus or tract. This is usually performed via a transverse neck incision. Platysma is divided and sternomastoid is retracted posteriorly to obtain access to the cyst. It is then removed by careful dissection with identification and by avoiding nerve damage (especially the vagus, hypoglossal and spinal accessory nerves). A branchial cyst abscess should first be drained and antibiotics given to eliminate infection before the cyst is excised.

COMPLICATIONS
Infection, branchial cyst abscess, nerve damage during surgery, incomplete excision of a sinus or fistula tract.

PROGNOSIS
Good, with cure following complete excision. Recurrence rates more common if previous infection.

Parathyroid disease

DEFINITION

Benign tumours of the parathyroid gland (parathyroid adenomas) or parathyroid hyperplasia with excessive parathyroid hormone (PTH) secretion, causing primary hyperparathyroidism with hypercalcaemia and osteomalacia.

Rarely, malignancy (parathyroid adenocarcinomas).

AETIOLOGY

The exact aetiology by which these benign tumours form is unknown. Previous radiation to head, neck and chest regions are associated with an increased likelihood of parathyroid adenomas.

Parathyroid adenomas may be part of an endocrine tumour syndrome (e.g. MENI and MENIIa).

EPIDEMIOLOGY

Uncommon. Approximately 1 per 1000; usually in 50–70 years of age.

HISTORY

Often asymptomatic and hypercalcaemia picked up on routine blood tests.
There may be symptoms of hypercalcaemia:

- Myalgia, arthralgia, fatigue
- Bone pain
- Nephrolithiasis
- Depression, anxiety, impaired consciousness
- Pancreatitis

EXAMINATION

There is normally nothing to find on examination other than the consequences of hypercalcaemia.

INVESTIGATIONS

Blood: U&E (to assess fluid balance and electrolytes), bone profile ($\uparrow$ Ca^{2+}, $\downarrow$ phosphate), $\uparrow$ plasma PTH.

Urine: Raised urinary calcium.

Plain radiographs: Osteopenia or osteoporosis. Cystic bone lesions.

CXR: To exclude sarcoidosis.

Nuclear imaging: Technetium-99 scintigraphy may identify the location of the adenoma.

US neck: Parathyroid adenomas can have distinct appearance.

DEXA bone scan: Necessary to assess the degree of osteopenia or osteoporosis.

MANAGEMENT

Treatment of hypercalcaemia: IV rehydration (normal saline). Once rehydrated, continue maintaining fluids with loop diuretics (e.g. furosemide) to enhance renal calcium excretion. Monitor other electrolytes. Consider IV pamidronate (increase bone resorption), calcitonin or steroids (but only effective in other causes of hypercalcaemia).

Surgery: Neck exploration and total parathyroidectomy (removal of all abnormal glands). If the site of the adenoma is clearly identified (requires >1 modality), directed parathyroidectomy may be an option; alternatively, parathyroidectomy guided by intraoperative monitoring of PTH levels can be performed as PTH levels drop within minutes after removal of the adenoma.

COMPLICATIONS

Risks of surgery:

- Post-operative hypoparathyroidism due to 'hungry bone syndrome' and may require short-term calcium and vitamin D supplementation.
- Recurrent laryngeal nerve injury is a serious risk, especially if the neck exploration is extensive. Laryngoscopy may detect vocal cord paralysis and an early operation to repair a transected nerve can reverse some of the injury.

■ Neck haematoma can compress the trachea compromising the airway; significant haematomas may require surgery to evacuate the haematoma.
Complications of hypercalcaemia, including nephrolithiasis, osteoporosis and cognitive
impairment.

PROGNOSIS
Good if the adenoma is entirely removed. Many patients do not need any additional
supplementation.

Salivary gland tumours

DEFINITION

Tumours arising in either the major (parotid, submandibular, sublingual) or minor salivary glands, characterised by a diversity of histological subtypes. Eighty per cent arise in the parotid (20% malignant); 15% in the submandibular (30–50% malignant); and 15% in the minor salivary glands (>60% malignant). Sublingual gland tumours are rare (0.3%, but nearly all malignant).

AETIOLOGY

Unknown cause. Please see **Associations/Risk Factors**.

ASSOCIATIONS/RISK FACTORS

Environmental factors identified: smoking (Warthin's), radiation (Warthin's and mucoepidermoid carcinoma); Epstein–Barr virus with lymphoepithelial tumours.

EPIDEMIOLOGY

Relatively rare, most occur in adults. Pleomorphic adenoma: mean age 42 years, Warthin's tumour: mean age 60 years (male > female); acinic cell carcinoma: affects women in 50s; squamous carcinomas: men in 70s.

HISTORY

A swelling, usually slow-growing and painless. Pain is more likely if the tumour is malignant.

EXAMINATION

The swelling should be examined with attention to evidence of fixation. In locally advanced cases, induration or ulceration of overlying skin or mucosa. The submandibular gland should be palpated bimanually. Inspection of the oral cavity as deep lobe parotid tumours may enlarge into the parapharyngeal space. Facial nerve function in parotid lesions (weakness should raise suspicion of malignancy) and evidence of regional lymphadenopathy.

INVESTIGATIONS

Imaging: Ultrasound, CT or MRI scanning is used in delineating the mass and its relationship to surrounding structures and staging.

Tissue biopsy: FNA can be used, but cannot absolutely be relied on for histological diagnosis. Incisional or excisional biopsy of masses in major glands should be avoided because of the risk of tumour spillage.

Histology:

- *Benign tumours*: Pleomorphic adenoma: 80–85% of parotid gland tumours. Epithelial or myoepithelial cells without a true capsule; hence propensity to recur after removal. Warthin's tumour (papillary cystadenoma lymphomatosum previously known as adenolymphoma): 15% of parotid neoplasms, 10% bilateral or multi-centric with glandular and cystic elements and eosinophilic epithelium.
- *Malignant carcinomas*: Acinic cell carcinoma: most commonly in parotid. Wide histological spectrum with lymphocytic infiltrates.
- *Mucoepidermoid carcinoma*: Most common malignant tumour of the parotid gland, of variable malignancy, i.e. low grade to aggressive.
- *Adenoid cystic carcinoma (6% most common malignant carcinoma of the submandibular)*: Aggressive with perineural spread into the brain and potential for late metastases.
- *Adenocarcinoma, squamous and undifferentiated carcinomas*: All aggressive.
- *Non-epithelial tumours (e.g. haemangiomas, lymphomas)*: All rare.

MANAGEMENT

Medical: Reserved for lymphoma or infective masses.

Surgical: Excision is used for both benign and malignant tumours.

Parotid: Superficial (for benign or low-grade malignancies) or total parotidectomy (for higher-grade malignancies) with careful preservation of the facial nerve and its branches that run between the deep and superficial lobes. If the nerve is involved, sacrifice and immediate reconstruction with a nerve graft can be performed.

Submandibular: Tumours are approached by an incision in the submandibular triangle. Malignant tumours may involve the lingual or hypoglossal nerves and resection may be necessary. This results in partial loss of sensation and movement of the tongue, this should be discussed with the patient. There is also a risk of injury to the mandibular branch of the facial nerve, resulting in asymmetry of the mouth/lower lip. Neck dissection is performed if lymph nodes are involved.

Carcinomas on the palate: Wide excision that may require complex reconstruction.

Radiotherapy: Adjuvant post-op radiotherapy should be given if malignant.

Chemotherapy: Not very successful, usually reserved for palliation.

COMPLICATIONS

Of parotidectomy: Facial nerve injury, haemorrhage, skin flap necrosis, salivary fistula and Frey's syndrome (10–50%, aberrant regeneration of postganglionic parasympathetic nerve fibres that normally innervate the parotid to sympathetic nerves of sweat glands, resulting in gustatory sweating). Pleomorphic adenomas have a high rate of recurrence if only simple enucleation is performed due to presence of pseudopod-like extensions from the tumour.

PROGNOSIS

Pleomorphic adenomas, if not removed, slowly enlarge and there is a risk of malignant transformation (5%). Mucoepidermoid carcinoma, 5-year survival is 70% (but worse for higher-grade forms). Adenoid cystic carcinoma has a poor prognosis (because perineural invasion is difficult to eradicate and has tendency for late recurrence). Low grade tumours 10-year survival is 80–95% but only 25–50% in high grade tumours.

Thyroglossal cyst and fistula

DEFINITION
Thyroglossal tract remnants found along the course of descent of the thyroid gland.

AETIOLOGY
The thyroglossal duct is a tract of embryonic mesoderm that originates between the first and second branchial pouches, represented by the foramen caecum of the tongue. It descends to a pretracheal site during development to form the thyroid gland. The duct normally disappears in the 6th week; however, if some tissue remains at any point along its course, it may develop into a cyst.
One to two per cent of cases are associated with lingual or ectopic thyroid tissue.

ASSOCIATIONS/RISK FACTORS
Please see **Aetiology.**

EPIDEMIOLOGY
Presents in children or adolescents, mean age of presentation is 5 years (but can vary from 4 months to 70 years). Three times more common than branchial cysts.

HISTORY
A swelling or lump is noticed in the midline of the anterior neck, mostly asymptomatic, but in 5% cases there may be tenderness or rapid enlargement due to infection.

EXAMINATION
Midline smooth rounded swelling (90%; 10% can be lateral, with 95% of these on the left side), typically between the thyroid notch and the hyoid bone, although sometimes found in the submental region.
Moves upwards on protrusion of the tongue and with swallowing and can usually be transilluminated.
Differential diagnosis: Lymph node, epidermal inclusion (dermoid) cysts, salivary duct abnormality or ectopic thyroid tissue.

PATHOLOGY/PATHOGENESIS
Thyroglossal cysts can occur at any point along the thyroglossal duct path, with 75% pre-hyoid. The lining is non-keratinising stratified squamous, columnar or cuboidal epithelium with mucoid material filling the cyst. Can contain ectopic thyroid tissue.

INVESTIGATIONS
Ultrasound or MRI scan: To differentiate from other structures (cysts have a high signal on T2 weighting).
Blood: Thyroid function tests.
Fine-needle aspiration cytology: Pre-operatively (usually benign epithelia, respiratory or squamous).

MANAGEMENT
Any acute infection is treated with antibiotics.
Surgical: Excision is carried out with the Sistrunk procedure (removal of the cyst and any duct remnant along with the central portion of the hyoid bone). Rarely, the tract may extend up to the tongue, requiring removal of a small portion of the tongue.

COMPLICATIONS
Infection is the most common complication. Thyroglossal sinus or fistula may develop after infection and spontaneous rupture, after attempted drainage or incomplete excision. Carcinoma in a thyroglossal duct cyst has rarely been described.

PROGNOSIS
Good, but even with good technique, recurrence rates are 7–8%, more commonly following infection.

Thyroid cancer

DEFINITION
Malignancy arising in the thyroid gland; types include papillary, follicular, medullary and anaplastic tumours.

AETIOLOGY
Please see **Associations/Risk Factors**.

ASSOCIATIONS/RISK FACTORS
Childhood exposure to radiation (papillary tumours). Associated with MAPK pathway and p53 gene mutations. Medullary thyroid carcinomas may be familial and are associated with MEN syndrome type IIa or IIb (20% cases). Lymphoma is associated with Hashimoto's thyroiditis.

EPIDEMIOLOGY
Commonest endocrine malignancy. Incidence is increasing 8.2/100,000. Female:male is 3:1. Age: papillary 20–40 years, follicular 40–50 years, and anaplastic tumours tend to occur in older age.

HISTORY
A slow-growing thyroid/neck lump/nodule.
The patient may complain of discomfort while swallowing or a hoarse voice.

EXAMINATION
Palpable nodule or diffuse enlargement of the thyroid. If cervical nodes are enlarged, malignancy should be suspected. The patient is usually euthyroid.

INVESTIGATIONS
Blood: TFT (if hyperthyroid, thyroid nodule is less likely to be malignant), bone profile, serum thyroglobulin (tumour marker for papillary and follicular tumours) and calcitonin (tumour marker for medullary carcinoma).
FNA cytology (FNAC) or ultrasound-guided core needle biopsy: Allows for histological diagnosis. Lymph node biopsy: If there is an enlarged cervical lymph node.
Imaging: Ultrasound, isotope scanning, CT and/or MRI staging, bone scan.
Histology:
- Papillary adenocarcinomas (70%) tend to be multi-focal, a characteristic is 'orphan Annie' pale, empty and grooved nuclei. They invade lymphatics with early spread.
- Follicular adenocarcinomas (15%) are encapsulated and undergo haematogenous spread to bone and lung. Follicular tumours cannot be diagnosed on FNAC as malignancy is based on vascular and/or capsular invasion.
- Medullary adenocarcinomas (5–10%) are well differentiated and derived from parafollicular calcitonin-secreting C cells.
- Anaplastic carcinomas are undifferenciated pleomorphic tumours, stain for cytokeratins and are very aggressive.
- Lymphomas are rare (2.5% of extra nodal lymphomas) and usually diffuse B cell.

MANAGEMENT
Surgical: Total thyroidectomy with block dissection of any affected lymph nodes. Subtotal thyroid lobectomy is possible for well-localised papillary tumours. Anaplastic tumours tend to be hard fixed masses and local debulking and tracheal compression may be the only option.
Medical: *Chemotherapy*: Thyroxine treatment to avoid hypothyroidism post-surgery and to suppress residual tumour cells in papillary and follicular tumours (which may be stimulated by TSH). Doxorubicin chemotherapy is used in anaplastic tumours.
Radiological: ^{131}I-radioiodine treatment for papillary tumour extending beyond the capsule, recurrences and metastasis. External radiotherapy for local recurrences. Anaplastic tumours are poorly responsive.

Thyroid cancer (continued)

COMPLICATIONS

From disease: Dysphonia, hoarseness due to recurrent laryngeal nerve involvement, airway obstruction, tracheomalacia from compression, dysphagia.

From surgery: Haemorrhage, recurrent laryngeal nerve damage, superior laryngeal nerve paresis, laryngeal oedema, hypoparathyroidism, hypothyroidism.

PROGNOSIS

Important factors are tumour type, size and stage. Papillary carcinomas have an overall 90% 10-year survival, best in those <40 years with tumours <1.5 cm; follicular have overall 85% 10-year survival; medullary have 5-year survival of 90% (node negative) and 50% (node positive), worse in men and those aged >50 years. Lymphomas confined within the capsule have an 85% 5-year survival, which drops to 40% with local spread. Anaplastic carcinomas have a very poor prognosis.

Thyroid goitre

DEFINITION
Abnormal enlargement of the thyroid gland. Can be diffuse or multi-nodular. Toxic or non-toxic.

AETIOLOGY
Non-toxic goitre: Often unknown. Linked to iodine deficiency (endemic goitre), iodine excess (rare). Goitrogens such as drugs, e.g. lithium, vegetables such as cabbage and sprouts. Toxic multi-nodular goitre (Plummer's disease) 15–30% of hyperthyroidism, Grave's disease.

ASSOCIATIONS/RISK FACTORS
Please see **Aetiology**.

EPIDEMIOLOGY
Sporadic non-toxic goitre, prevalence up to 8.5% of UK population. Women:men is 4:1.

HISTORY
Most asymptomatic and noticed as a swelling in the neck. Occasionally, tightness, cough, hoarseness, rarely dysphagia or dyspnoea. Symptoms of hyperthyroidism or hypothyroidism.

EXAMINATION
Consistency of the thyroid may be smooth or multi-nodular.
The swelling may extend to the superior mediastinum.
Check for tracheal deviation and lymphadenopathy.
Hypervascular thyrotoxic goitre may have a bruit.
Check for signs of thyroid status and thyroid eye disease.

PATHOLOGY/PATHOGENESIS
Diffuse follicular epithelial hyperplasia. With time follicles may coalesce to form nodules, with areas of involution, fibrosis and cyst formation.

INVESTIGATIONS
Blood: Thyroid function tests, thyroid antibodies.
Ultrasound: Differentiate between diffuse, multi-nodular and solitary nodule.
Radiology: Chest radiograph to check for retrosternal extension. CT or MRI if surgery is planned and there is a large retrosternal component.
Laryngoscopy: Visualisation of vocal cord prior to any surgery to document any vocal cord palsy.
Cytology: FNA if there is a solitary nodule
Radioiodine isotope scan: To determine if a nodule is functioning (hot) or non-functioning (cold). Ninety-nine per cent hot nodules are benign.

MANAGEMENT
Conservative: Prevention in endemic areas by adding iodine to water supply. Non-toxic goitres often do not need surgical treatment unless causing symptoms or if concern about a specific nodule.
Medical: Correction of thyroid status. Radioactive iodine (^{131}I) therapy reduces thyroid volume by 50–60%, usually in older patients in whom surgery is higher risk.
Surgical: Indications are compressive symptoms, risk of malignancy or cosmetic deformity. Subtotal or total thyroidectomy is performed.

COMPLICATIONS
If large: Goitre can cause compression of neck structures.
Of surgery: Recurrent laryngeal nerve damage, parathyroid gland excision leading to hypocalcaemia; post-operative haemorrhage is an emergency requiring immediate decompression of the wound.

PROGNOSIS
Generally good, as usually non-toxic goitres grow slowly over years. If growth is rapid, malignancy should be excluded.

Cholangiocarcinoma

DEFINITION
Epithelial cancer arising from bile ducts.

AETIOLOGY
Associated with chronic inflammation and cholestasis: Primary sclerosing cholangitis (1.5% cumulative annual risk), choledochal cysts, Caroli's disease and congenital hepatic fibrosis, parasitic infections of the biliary tract (e.g. *Clonorchis sinensis*, liver flukes), hepatolithiasis, Thorotrast (contrast agent used in the 1930s to 1950s), Lynch syndrome II, biliary papillomatosis.

EPIDEMIOLOGY
Uncommon (0.3–0.6% of cancer deaths), but increasing in incidence (has now overtaken hepatocellular carcinoma as the most common cause of mortality from primary liver tumours in England). Highest rates in Asia (due to parasitic infection). Slightly more common in males.

HISTORY
Obstructive jaundice (yellow skin and sclera, pale stools, dark urine, pruritus).
Abdominal fullness or pain.
Symptoms of malignancy: weight loss, fatigue, malaise.

EXAMINATION
Jaundice. Palpable gallbladder (Courvoisier's law states that, in the presence of jaundice, an enlarged gallbladder is unlikely to be due to gallstones; i.e. carcinoma of the pancreas or the lower biliary tree is more likely).
Epigastric or right upper quadrant mass in advanced cases.

PATHOLOGY/PATHOGENESIS
Described according to location as intrahepatic (10%) or extrahepatic [90%, hilar (Klatskin tumours), mid-duct, distal and diffuse]. Bismuth classification of hilar tumours into types I–V based on their location in relation to the confluence of hepatic ducts. Three different growth patterns of extrahepatic types: mass forming, periductal infiltrating and intraductal growing.

INVESTIGATIONS
Blood: FBC, U&Es, LFTs, clotting, tumour markers (CA19-9, CEA often raised, but are not specific).
Endoscopy: ERCP/Endoscopic ultrasound enables bile cytology, tumour biopsy if accessible and interventions to relieve obstructive jaundice. Percutaneous transhepatic cholangiography (PTC) is an alternative in cases of difficult bile duct access.
Ultrasound: Variable sensitivity but will show biliary duct dilation.
CT, MRI or MRCP, PET scan: To stage tumour and visualise any regional spread.
Arteriogram (invasive or MR): Important when considering surgery to show any involvement of surrounding vascular structures.
Staging: TNM staging.

MANAGEMENT
Medical: Palliative measures in unresectable tumours. Endoscopic (or percutaneous) biliary decompression by insertion of plastic or metal stents; the latter have higher patency rates.
Chemo/Radiotherapy: Intracavity or brachytherapy can reduce tumour size; however, chemotherapy response rates are poor at present. Photodynamic therapy has been shown to palliate symptoms and may improve survival.
Surgical: The only curative treatment but <15% are resectable. Solitary intrahepatic tumours: segmentectomy or lobectomy. Portal vein embolisation followed by extended hepatectomy for hilar tumours. Distal tumours: Whipple's procedure (proximal pancreaticoduodenectomy with choledocho- or hepaticojejunostomy). Resection should be with curative intent as there

Cholangiocarcinoma (continued)

is no significant survival benefit in non-curative/debulking surgery. Results of liver transplantation are poor.

COMPLICATIONS

Obstructive jaundice, cholangitis, metastases (lymphatic or local hepatic spread are usual routes).

PROGNOSIS

Poor, median survival <24 months. Five-year survival rate following resection is ~40%.

Gallbladder cancer

DEFINITION
Malignancy arising from the gallbladder.

AETIOLOGY
Gallstone disease (80% of patients; however, only 0.3–3% with stones will develop the disease). A 'porcelain gallbladder', so called because of mural calcification (up to 60%). Gallbladder polyps (>10 mm) and anomalous pancreaticobiliary anatomy.

EPIDEMIOLOGY
Most common biliary tract malignancy, 5th most common GI malignancy, age usually >65 years. Female:male ratio is 2–3:1.

HISTORY
Early may be discovered on investigation for gallstone disease. When symptoms are present, e.g. abdominal fullness, pain and weight loss, the disease often advanced.

EXAMINATION
A palpable right upper quadrant mass may be present. Signs of weight loss. Jaundice.

PATHOLOGY/PATHOGENESIS
Ninety per cent are adenocarcinomas, 5% squamous carcinomas and 5% anaplastic carcinomas. Thickening, induration or mass in the fundus (60%), body (30%) or neck (5%).

INVESTIGATIONS
Ultrasound: May show gallbladder wall thickening, polyp or a mass, sensitivity ~85%, colour Doppler may improve specificity.
CT, MRI, MRA, MRCP: To assess tumour and examine for metastases.
Others: FDG-PET, ERCP or PTC in biliary obstruction, laparoscopy.
Tumour markers: CEA, CA19-9 and CA125 can be raised.

MANAGEMENT
Surgical: Simple cholecystectomy for tumours confined to the mucosa or submucosa (T1a). For tumours invading the muscularis, radical cholecystectomy with hepatic wedge resection (segments IV, V, at least 3 cm in depth), resection of the cystic duct and regional lymph nodes. If pericholedochal nodes are involved, the common bile duct may be resected with restoration of biliary-enteric continuity with a Roux-en-Y hepaticojejunostomy.
Chemotherapy or radiotherapy: Some agents have partial responses (e.g. 5-fluorouracil). Radiotherapy is also used.
Palliative: Obstructive jaundice can be managed with endoscopic or percutaneous stenting. Pain relief is a prime concern, and may be helped by percutaneous coeliac nerve block or chemical splanchnicectomy. Responds poorly to chemotherapy and radiotherapy.

COMPLICATIONS
Obstructive jaundice, pain, duodenal obstruction.
Spread: Local direct invasion into the hepatic bed (venous drainage into segment IV), lymphatic spread into the cystic, pancreaticoduodenal, coeliac and periaortic nodes. Transperitoneal spread is also common.

PROGNOSIS
With the exception of cases detected incidentally at cholecystectomy, prognosis is poor and all stage 5-year survival ~5%.
Staging: TNM, based on the depth of invasion, correlates with prognosis.

Gallstones

DEFINITION
Stone formation in the gallbladder.

AETIOLOGY
- *Mixed stones:* Contain cholesterol, calcium bilirubinate, phosphate and protein (80%). Associated with older age, female, obesity, parenteral nutrition, drugs (OCP, octreotide), family history, ethnicity (e.g. Pima Indians), interruption of the enterohepatic recirculation of bile salts (e.g. Crohn's disease), terminal ileal resection.
- *Pure cholesterol stones (10%):* Similar associations with mixed stones.
- *Pigment stones (10%):* Black stones made of calcium bilirubinate: (↑ bilirubin 2° to haemolytic disorders e.g. sickle cell, cirrhosis), brown stones due to bile duct infestation by liver fluke *Clonorchis sinensis*.

EPIDEMIOLOGY
Very common (UK prevalence ~10%), more common with age, 3× more females in younger population but equal sex ratio after 65 years. About 50,000 cholecystectomies are performed annually in the UK.

HISTORY
Asymptomatic (90%): found incidentally.
Biliary colic: Sudden onset, severe right upper quadrant or epigastric pain, constant in nature. May radiate to right scapula, often precipitated by a fatty meal. May be associated with nausea and vomiting.
Acute cholecystitis: Patient systemically unwell, fever, prolonged upper abdominal pain that may be referred to the right shoulder (due to diaphragmatic irritation).
Ascending cholangitis: Classical association between right upper quadrant pain, jaundice and rigors (Charcot's triad). If combined with hypotension and confusion, it is known as Reynold's pentad.

EXAMINATION
Biliary colic: Right upper quadrant or epigastric tenderness.
Acute cholecystitis: Tachycardia, pyrexia, right upper quadrant or epigastric tenderness. There may be guarding ± rebound. Positive Murphy's sign.
Ascending cholangitis: Pyrexia, right upper quadrant pain, jaundice.

PATHOLOGY/PATHOGENESIS
Biliary colic is caused by impaction of a gallstone in the cystic duct. Resolves when stone falls back into gallbladder, or stone remains impacted leading to inflammation and mucosal oedema and acute cholecystitis. In chronic cholecystitis, the pathological changes vary from microscopic evidence of chronic inflammation with the mucosa penetrating the muscle layer as Rokitansky–Aschoff sinuses to a shrunken fibrosed gallbladder with transmural fibrosis. Rarely, dystrophic calcification occurs resulting in a 'porcelain gallbladder', with ↑ risk of malignant transformation.

INVESTIGATIONS
Blood: FBC (↑ WBC in cholecystitis or cholangitis), LFT (↑ AlkPhos, ↑ bilirubin in ascending cholangitis. There may be ↑ transaminases), blood cultures, amylase (risk of pancreatitis).
USS: Demonstrates gallstones (acoustic shadow within the gallbladder) and ↑ thickness of gallbladder wall, and can examine for presence of dilatation of biliary tree indicative of obstruction. AXR: Gallstones are infrequently radio-opaque (10%) (see Fig. 5).
Other imaging: Erect CXR (to exclude perforation as a differential diagnosis, CT scanning, MRCP or ERCP.

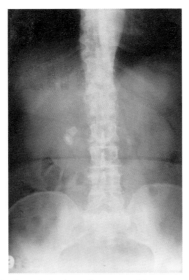

Figure 5 Plain abdominal radiograph showing radio-opaque gallstones.

MANAGEMENT
Conservative: For mild symptoms of biliary colic, avoidance of fat in diet.
Medical: Oral dissolution therapy is poorly effective, slow and has a high recurrence rate, only suitable for a small number of patients. If biliary colic is severe, this may require admission, IV fluids with analgesia and antiemetics; if there are signs of infection, antibiotics should be prescribed. If symptoms fail to improve or worsen, a localised abscess or empyema should be suspected. This can be drained percutaneously by cholecystostomy and pigtail catheter. If there is ascending cholangitis, resuscitation and IV antibiotics. If there is obstruction, urgent biliary drainage by ERCP or PTC.
Surgical: Laparoscopic cholecystectomy (see Cholecystectomy) ± on table cholangiogram. In acute setting, should be performed within 72 hours of symptom onset of 'hot gallbladder', or after several weeks to allow inflammation to settle.

COMPLICATIONS
Stones within gallbladder: Biliary colic, cholecystitis, mucocoele or gallbladder empyema, porcelain gallbladder, predisposition to gallbladder cancer (rare).
Stones outside gallbladder: Obstructive jaundice, pancreatitis, ascending cholangitis, perforation and pericholecystic abscess or bile peritonitis, cholecystenteric fistula, gallstone ileus, Bouveret's syndrome (gallstones causing gastric outlet obstruction), cholecystocholedochal fistula (Mirizzi's syndrome).
Of cholecystectomy: Bleeding, infection, bile leak, bile duct injury (0.3%), post-cholecystectomy syndrome (persistant dyspeptic symptoms), hernias.

PROGNOSIS
In most cases, gallstones are benign and do not cause significant problems (2% with gallstones develop symptoms annually). If symptomatic, surgery is an effective treatment.

Hepatocellular carcinoma

DEFINITION
Primary malignancy of the liver parenchyma.

AETIOLOGY
- Chronic liver damage – 1–6% cirrhosis per year. Hepatitis B and C and haemochromatosis highest risk.
- Aflatoxins (from cereals contaminated with fungi or biological weapons).

EPIDEMIOLOGY
Fourth most common cancer worldwide, 1 million deaths per year. Less common than secondary liver malignancies. ↑ incidence in regions where hepatitis B and C are endemic (e.g. southern Mediterranean, Far East).

HISTORY
History of malignancy: Malaise, weight loss, loss of appetite.
History of liver cirrhosis: Fullness in abdomen and jaundice are often the only symptoms.

EXAMINATION
Signs of malignancy: Cachexia, lymphadenopathy.
Hepatomegaly: Nodular (but may be smooth).
Deep palpation may elicit tenderness.
Jaundice, ascites.
There may be bruit heard over the liver.

INVESTIGATION
Blood: FBC, ESR, LFT, clotting, α-fetoprotein, hepatitis serology.
Imaging: Abdominal ultrasound may identify a lesion within a cirrhotic liver. CT scan or MRI is the gold standard for staging.
Angiography: If transarterial embolisation is being considered.
Histology: Ascites may be aspirated and sent for cytology.
Staging: Chest, abdomen and pelvic CT scans. Consider bone scan.

MANAGEMENT
Medical: Chemotherapy, transarterial chemoembolisation, newer agents that may have increased response include tyrosine kinase inhibitors, e.g. sorafenib.
Surgical: Liver resection is indicated if localised to a single lobe. Liver transplantation can be considered. Criteria for transplantation are the 'Milan criteria', i.e. one tumour <5 cm or <3 tumours <3 cm.
Radiotherapy: Radioembolisation, e.g. Yttrium-90 microspheres.
Ablation: Useful to shrink tumours not amenable to resection. Radiofrequency, cryoablation, or percutaneous ethanol injection are used.

COMPLICATIONS
Biliary tree obstruction, acute liver failure, hepatic rupture and haemoperitoneum, reactive pleural effusion, distant metastases.

PROGNOSIS
Very poor. Majority of patients die within 1 year of diagnosis, and surgical cure is only possible in ~5%.

Liver abscess

DEFINITION
Infection resulting in a walled-off collection of pus in the liver.

AETIOLOGY
Pyogenic (80–85%): *Escherichia coli*, *Klebsiellae*, enterococci, *Bacteroides*, streptococci, staphylococci. Usually arise from biliary tract sepsis or other source drained by the portal circulation, e.g. appendicitis. Less commonly associated with tumours, post-hepatic embolisation or penetrating liver trauma. In children, may be associated with underlying immune deficiency.
Amoebic: Secondary infection from amoebic gut infection (*Entamoeba histolytica*). Abscesses contain 'anchovy sauce' fluid of necrotic hepatocytes and trophozoites.
Hydatid: Tapeworm, *Echinococcus granulosis*. Grow slowly, can hold litres of fluid, produce tissue damage by mechanical pressure and contain millions of infective stages, which are called hydatid sand (brood capsules and protoscolices).
Fungal: *Candida albicans*, *Aspergillus*. Associated with prolonged exposure to antibiotics, transplantation and immunosuppression or immunodeficiency.

EPIDEMIOLOGY
Pyogenic: Annual incidence is 0.8/100,000. Mean age is 60 years, most common type in the developed world.
Amoebic: Most common type worldwide.
Hydatid: More common in sheep-rearing countries.

HISTORY
Fever, malaise, anorexia, night sweats, weight loss, hiccups due to diaphragmatic irritation.
Right upper quadrant or epigastric pain, which may be referred to shoulder (diaphragmatic irritation).
Jaundice, diarrhoea, pyrexia of unknown origin.

EXAMINATION
Fever (continuous or spiking), jaundice (due to biliary tract pathology or multiple abscesses). Tender hepatomegaly, occasionally signs of a reactive pleural effusion or atelectasis on the right.

INVESTIGATIONS
Blood: FBC (mild anaemia, leukocytosis, ↑ eosinophils in hydatid disease), LFT (↑ AlkPhos, ↑ bilirubin), ↑ ESR, ↑ CRP, blood cultures, amoebic and hydatid serology.
Stool microscopy, cultures: May pick up *E. histolytica* or tapeworm eggs.
Ultrasound: Hypoechoic lesions with possible internal septations or debris, also allows biliary tract assessment and guides aspiration.
CT: Abscesses are typically hypodense with peripheral contrast enhancement.
CXR: Right pleural effusion or atelectasis, raised hemidiaphragm.
Aspiration: For diagnosis and treatment.

MANAGEMENT
Pyogenic/Fungal: Percutaneous (under ultrasound or CT guidance) aspiration (if small-sized) or catheter drainage (if moderate size) or occasionally surgical drainage (if large or multi-locular abscesses). Broad-spectrum antibiotics or antifungals. Treatment of underlying cause.
Amoebic: Metronidazole followed by treatment with a luminal amoebicide, e.g. diloxanide furoate.
Hydatid: Surgical removal (pericystectomy) with mebendazole or albendazole treatment to reduce risk recurrence. The PAIR technique involves puncture, aspiration, injection and reaspiration. In inoperable cases, drugs can be used.

Liver abscess (continued)

COMPLICATIONS

Septic shock, rupture and dissemination (e.g. into biliary tract causing acute cholangitis, intrathoracic rupture or peritonitis), allergic sequelae or anaphylaxis from ruptured hydatid cyst.

PROGNOSIS

Untreated pyogenic liver abscesses often fatal; complications have high mortality. Amoebic abscesses have a better prognosis and usually have a quick response to therapy; hydatid cysts may recur after surgery (10%).

Pancreatic cancer

DEFINITION
Malignancy arising from the exocrine or endocrine tissues of the pancreas.

AETIOLOGY
Unknown cause. Five to 10 per cent have a familial component, and hereditary syndromes include BRCA-2 mutation, Familial atypical multiple mole melanoma (CDKN2A), Peutz–Jeghers (STK11/LKB1), hereditary pancreatitis (PRSS1), MEN, HNPCC, FAP, Gardner, von Hippel–Lindau syndromes. Precursor lesions include pancreatic intraductal neoplasia, intraductal pancreatic mucinous neoplasm and mucinous cystic neoplasm.

EPIDEMIOLOGY
Increasing in incidence (8–12/100,000), worldwide 8th cause of cancer deaths. Two times more males, peak age 60–80 years.

HISTORY
Clinical diagnosis of pancreatic cancer is often difficult as the initial symptoms are often quite non-specific. These include anorexia, malaise, weight loss, nausea. Later, jaundice, epigastric pain.

EXAMINATION
Signs of weight loss, epigastric tenderness or mass.
Jaundice and a palpable gallbladder (Courvoisier's law).*
In patients with metastatic spread, there may be hepatomegaly.
Trousseau's sign is an associated superficial thrombophlebitis.

PATHOLOGY/PATHOGENESIS
Seventy-five per cent occur within the head or neck of the pancreas (where it can present as a periampullary tumour), 15–20% occur in the body and 5–10% occur in the tail. Spread is local and to the liver. Eighty per cent are adenocarcinomas, and other types include adenosquamous and mucinous cystadenocarcinomas. Endocrine tumours include insulinomas, glucagonomas and gastrinomas.

INVESTIGATIONS
Bloods: Tumour markers CA19-9 and CEA can be elevated (former more specific, but neither are diagnostic). If causing obstructive jaundice, ↑ bilirubin, ↑ ALP, clotting may be deranged.
Imaging: Ultrasound, endoscopic ultrasound and FNA, CT, MRI, PET and laparoscopy are all useful in staging the disease. ERCP may allow biopsy/bile cytology ± stenting.
Other: Staging laparoscopy or intraoperative ultrasound.

MANAGEMENT
Medical: Most patients with disease who are not amenable to curative resection undergo palliative management. This may involve chemotherapy, e.g. gemcitabine, cisplatin or the epidermal growth factor receptor antagonist, erlotinib. Pain relief by medical analgesia, radiotherapy or coeliac plexus block. For obstructive jaundice, endoscopic stent insertion or a surgical choledochojejunostomy. For duodenal obstruction, endoscopic stenting or a gastrojejunostomy.
Surgery: Only ~20% of patients are suitable; tumours on the body and tail are often unresectable at presentation.
Pancreaticoduodenectomy (Whipple procedure, See page 184): For tumours of the head (no vascular involvement or metastases). Involves *en bloc* resection of the pancreatic

*Courvoisier's law: Palpable gallbladder with painless jaundice is unlikely to be caused by gallstones.

Pancreatic cancer (continued)

head, first to third parts of the duodenum; the distal antrum; and the distal common bile duct. The GI tract is reconstructed with a gastrojejunostomy. The common bile duct and residual pancreas are anastomosed into a segment of small bowel.

Pylorus-preserving pancreaticoduodenectomy: Sparing the pylorus allows for more physiological emptying of the stomach.

COMPLICATIONS

Unresectable disease, pain, obstructive jaundice, pruritus, cholangitis, diabetes, splenic vein thrombosis, malignant ascites.

From surgery: Anastomotic leaks, bleeding, collections, pancreatic fistulas, brittle diabetes.

PROGNOSIS

Fewer than 5% of all patients are alive at 5 years. The median survival of all patients after initial diagnosis is 4–6 months. In patients able to undergo a successful curative resection, the median survival ranges from 12 to 19 months, and the 5-year survival rate is 15–20%. Patients with periampullary and endocrine tumours have a better prognosis.

Pancreatitis, acute

DEFINITION

An acute inflammatory process of the pancreas with variable involvement of other regional tissues or remote organ systems.

Mild: Associated with minimal organ dysfunction and uneventful recovery.

Severe: Associated with organ failure and/or local complications such as necrosis, abscess or pseudocyst (1992 Atlanta Classification).

AETIOLOGY

Insult results in activation of pancreatic proenzymes within the ducts/acini, resulting in tissue damage and inflammation.

Most common: Gallstones, alcohol (80% cases).

Others: Drugs (e.g. steroids, azathioprine, thiazides, valproate), trauma, ERCP or abdominal surgery, infective (e.g. mumps, EBV, CMV, Coxsackie B, mycoplasma), hyperlipidaemia, hyperparathyroidism, anatomical (e.g. pancreas divisum, annular pancreas), idiopathic.

EPIDEMIOLOGY

Common. Annual UK incidence ~10/10,000. Peak age is 60 years; in males, alcohol-induced disease is more common while in females, the principal cause is gallstones.

HISTORY

Severe epigastric or abdominal pain (radiating to back, relieved by sitting forward, aggravated by movement).

Associated with anorexia, nausea and vomiting.

There may be a history of gallstones or alcohol intake.

EXAMINATION

Epigastric tenderness, fever. Shock, tachycardia, tachypnoea.

↓ bowel sounds (due to ileus).

If severe and haemorrhagic, Turner's sign (flank bruising) or Cullen's sign (periumbilical bruising).

INVESTIGATIONS

Bloods: ↑ Amylase (usually >3× normal but does not correlate with severity), ↑ lipase, FBC (↑ WCC), U&Es, ↑ glucose, ↑ CRP, ↓ Ca^{2+}, LFTs (may be deranged if gallstone pancreatitis or alcohol), ABG (for hypoxia or metabolic acidosis).

USS: For gallstones or biliary dilatation.

Erect CXR: There may be pleural effusion. Mainly for excluding other causes.

AXR: To exclude other causes of acute abdomen. Psoas shadow may be lost.

CT scan: If diagnostic uncertainty or if persisting organ failure, signs of sepsis, necrosis or deterioration. Scoring system (Balthazar score): combination of the grade of pancreatitis and the degree of necrosis.

MANAGEMENT

Assessment of severity: The two most validated scales are the following:

1. Modified Glasgow criteria*combined with CRP (>220 mg/L)
2. APACHE-II score (see Gut 1998;**42**(Suppl 2):S1–S13).

Alternatively, there is Ranson's criteria.[†]

*Modified Glasgow criteria (≥3 indicates severe disease):

(**P**) $pO_2 < 8$ kPa	(u**R**) Urea > 16 mmol/L
(**A**) Age > 55	(**E**nz) LDH > 600 units/L
(**N**) WCC > 15 × 10^9/L	(**A**) Albumin < 32 g/L
(**C**) $Ca^{2+} < 2$ mmol/L	(**S**ugar) Glucose > 10 mmol/L

[†]*Ranson's criteria (only for alcoholic pancreatitis):*

On admission: WCC > 16 × 10^9/L, age >55, AST >250, LDH >350, glucose >11 mmol/L.

During first 48 hours: $pO_2 < 8$ kPa, $Ca^{2+} < 2$ mmol/L, urea >16 mmol/L, base deficit >4, haematocrit fall >10%, fluid sequestration >600 ml.

Pancreatitis, acute (continued)

Medical: Fluid and electrolyte resuscitation, urinary catheter and NG tube if vomiting. Analgesia and blood sugar control. Early HDU or intensive care support if severe. Meta-analysis has shown reduced infective complications and mortality in severe pancreatitis with enteral, as opposed to parenteral, feeding. Prophylactic antibiotics have not been shown to reduce mortality, unless infected pancreatic necrosis develops.

ERCP and sphincterotomy: For gallstone pancreatitis, cholangitis, jaundice or dilated common bile duct, ideally within 72 hours. All patients should undergo definitive management of gallstones during same admission or within 2 weeks.

Early detection and treatment of complications: For example, if persistent symptoms and >30% pancreatic necrosis or signs of sepsis, should undergo image-guided fine-needle aspiration for culture (BSG guidelines).

Surgical: Patient with necrotising pancreatitis should be managed in a specialist unit. Minimal access or open necrosectomy (drainage and debridement of all necrotic tissue).

COMPLICATIONS

Local: Pancreatic necrosis, pseudocyst (peripancreatic fluid collection persisting >4 weeks), abscess, ascites, pseudo-aneurysm or venous thrombosis.

Systemic: Multi-organ dysfunction, sepsis, renal failure, ARDS, DIC, hypocalcaemia, diabetes.

Long term: Chronic pancreatitis (with diabetes and malabsorption).

PROGNOSIS

Twenty per cent follow severe fulminating course with high mortality (infected pancreatic necrosis associated with 70% mortality), and 80% run milder course (but still 5% mortality).

Pancreatitis, chronic

DEFINITION

Chronic inflammatory disease of the pancreas characterised by irreversible parenchymal atrophy and fibrosis leading to impaired endocrine and exocrine function and recurrent abdominal pain.

AETIOLOGY

Alcohol (70%). Idiopathic in 20%.

Rare: Recurrent acute pancreatitis, ductal obstruction, pancreas divisum, hereditary pancreatitis, tropical pancreatitis, autoimmune pancreatitis, hyperparathyroidism, hypertriglyceridemia.

EPIDEMIOLOGY

Annual UK incidence ~1/100,000; prevalence ~3/100,000. Mean age 40–50 years in alcohol-associated disease.

HISTORY

Recurrent severe epigastric pain, radiating to back, relieved by sitting forward, can be exacerbated by eating or drinking alcohol. Over many years, weight loss, bloating and pale offensive stools (steatorrhoea).

EXAMINATION

Epigastric tenderness. Signs of complications, e.g. weight loss, malnutrition.

PATHOLOGY/PATHOGENESIS

Disruption of normal pancreatic glandular architecture due to chronic inflammation and fibrosis, calcification, parenchymal atrophy, ductal dilatation, cyst and stone formation. Pancreatic stellate cells are thought to play a role, converting from quiescent fat-storing cells to myofibroblast-like cells forming extracellular matrix, cytokines and growth factors in response to injury. Pain is associated with raised intraductal pressures and inflammation.

INVESTIGATIONS

Blood: Glucose ($\uparrow$ may indicate endocrine dysfunction), glucose tolerance test. Amylase and lipase (usually normal), $\uparrow$ immunoglobulins, especially IgG_4 in autoimmune pancreatitis.
USS: Percutaneous or endoscopic: can show hyperechoic foci with post-acoustic shadowing.
ERCP or MRCP: Early changes include main duct dilatation and stumping of branches. Late manifestations are duct strictures with alternating dilatation ('chain of lakes' appearance).
AXR: Pancreatic calcification may be visible (see Fig. 6).
CT scan: Pancreatic cysts, calcification.
Tests of pancreatic exocrine function: Faecal elastase.

MANAGEMENT

General: Treatment is mainly symptomatic and supportive, e.g. dietary advice, abstinence from alcohol and smoking, treatment of diabetes, oral pancreatic enzyme replacements, e.g. Creon, analgesia for exacerbations of pain. Chronic pain management may need specialist input. The sensory nerves to the pancreas transverse the coeliac ganglia and splanchnic nerves; coeliac plexus block (CT or EUS-guided neurolysis) and transthoracic splanchnicectomy offer variable degrees of pain relief.
Endoscopic therapy: Sphincterotomy, stone extraction, dilatation or stenting of strictures. Extracorporeal shock-wave lithotripsy is sometimes used for fragmentation of larger pancreatic stones prior to endoscopic removal.
Surgical: May be indicated if medical management has failed. Options include lateral pancreaticojejunal drainage (modified Puestow procedure), resection (pancreaticoduodenectomy or Whipple's) or limited resection of the pancreatic head (Beger procedure) or combined opening of the pancreatic duct and excavation of the pancreatic head (Frey procedure).

Pancreatitis, chronic (continued)

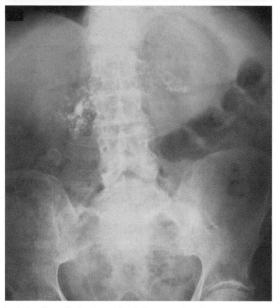

Figure 6 Abdominal radiograph showing with calcification within the pancreas indicative of chronic pancreatitis.

COMPLICATIONS
Local: Pseudocysts, biliary duct stricture, duodenal obstruction, pancreatic ascites, pancreatic carcinoma.
Systemic: Diabetes, steatorrhoea, reduced quality of life, chronic pain syndromes and dependence on strong analgesics.

PROGNOSIS
Difficult to predict as pain may improve, stabilize or worsen. Surgery improves symptoms in 60–70% but results are often not sustained. Life expectancy can be reduced by 10–20 years.

Anal carcinoma

DEFINITION

Malignancy arising in the anal canal or anal verge.

ASSOCIATIONS/RISK FACTORS

Linked to oncogenic types of human papilloma virus (e.g. 16, 18). Age >50 years. Genital warts, multiple sexual partners, homosexual men and those engaging in anoreceptive intercourse may be at higher risk, HIV or immunosuppressant drugs, chronic fistulae and previous pelvic irradiation may also ↑ risk as does smoking, although increased risk diminishes with smoking cessation.

EPIDEMIOLOGY

Uncommon, 3–4% of large bowel carcinomas, females>males (but anal margin tumours more common in men), mean age 50–70 years. Rising incidence.

HISTORY

Bleeding, pruritus ani, anal discomfort, pain or discharge, tenesmus, mass felt on the anal margin. If sphincter involvement, faecal incontinence. No symptoms.

EXAMINATION

An ulcer or proliferative growth may be seen on inspection of the anal margin or an area of induration or mass felt on PR examination. Fifteen to 30 per cent will have palpable inguinal lymph nodes at presentation (but only ~50% of these will contain tumour).

PATHOLOGY/PATHOGENESIS

Most common type is squamous cell carcinoma (80%), adenocarcinoma or rarely malignant melanoma (most common site after skin and eye), and are usually unpigmented. Anal intraepithelial neoplasia describes dysplasia in the squamous epithelium and is thought to be pre-malignant.

Anal carcinoma is classified based on location:

- Anal canal tumours (tend to be poorly differentiated non-keratinising)
- Anal margin tumours (15–30%, tend to be well differentiated producing keratin)

Tumours above the dentate line spread to pelvic lymph nodes, while those below spread to inguinal nodes.

INVESTIGATIONS

Proctoscopy and biopsy: For histology. Examination under anaesthesia may be necessary.
Blood: FBC (for anaemia), LFT.
Imaging: Endoanal ultrasound to assess invasion, MRI and CT, PET scan for staging.
TNM staging system: T0: no evidence of primary tumour; Tis: carcinoma in situ; T1: ≤2 cm, T2: ≥2 cm, < 5 cm; T3 > 5 cm; T4: any size but is growing into the surrounding tissues. N0: no lymph nodes; N1: perirectal lymph nodes involved; N2: unilateral pelvic or inguinal node involvement; N3: perirectal + pelvis or groin nodes or bilateral pelvis or groin nodes involved. Nx: regional nodes unassessed. Mx: metastasis unassessed; M0: no distant spread; M1: metastatic to distant organs or abdominal lymph nodes.

MANAGEMENT

Prevention: Minimise risk factors. There is a vaccine for HPV 16 and 18, although at present, this is only licenced for use in the prevention of cervical cancer. Future studies are planned for the use of the vaccine in the prevention of anal cancer.
Chemotherapy and radiotherapy: Agents (e.g. 5-fluorouracil and mitomicin C or cisplatin) are used in combination with local radiotherapy to the anal area and inguinal nodes. Outcomes comparable to radical surgery with preservation of the anal sphincter.

Anal carcinoma (continued)

Surgery: Local excision of small epidermoid carcinomas of the anal margin may be curative. In the past, abdominoperineal resection was carried out for carcinomas of the anal canal; however, with advances in chemoradiotherapy, this is now usually reserved for residual disease, recurrence post radiotherapy, those with obstructive cancers or other malignancies of the anal canal (e.g. adenocarcinoma).

COMPLICATIONS

Local: Pain, bleeding, incontinence, rectovaginal fistula if neglected.

From radiotherapy: Radiation-induced dermatitis, perineal irritation, proctitis and diarrhoea.

PROGNOSIS

Important factors are histological type, site, differentiation and stage. Five-year survival for early stage squamous carcinomas treated by radical chemo/radiotherapy is 80%; if inguinal nodes are involved, this is reduced to 30%. Melanoma in this region has a poor prognosis, with only a 10% cure rate by surgery.

Anal fissure

DEFINITION
An elongated ulcer in the long axis of the lower anal canal. 'Fissure-in-ano'.

AETIOLOGY
- *Traumatic*: Constipation: straining and passing hard stool tears the posterior anal lining. In women, anterior fissures are more common after childbirth when a damaged pelvic floor leaves the anterior anal tissues with less support.
- *Inflammatory*: Crohn's disease, ulcerative colitis.

EPIDEMIOLOGY
Most common under the age of 40. Incidence $\sim$1 : 350, male = female.

HISTORY
Severe burning pain on defaecation. Pain may persist for hours and may result in patients trying to avoid bowel movements. Bleeding per rectum is a common feature, is usually bright red, small in volume, on paper. There may be an associated pruritis ani.

EXAMINATION
Inspection often reveals a sentinel pile. Gentle traction on the anal skin can reveal the distal part of the fissure. Digital rectal examination may not be possible due to pain. In chronic fissures, it may be possible to feel a firm indurated ridge.

PATHOLOGY/PATHOGENESIS
A mechanical tear occurs in the anal mucosa and the underlying sphincter muscle goes into spasm. The spasm is not only painful but also perpetuates the problem by pulling the edges of the tear apart. The blood flow in the posterior midline of the anoderm is less than in other parts of the anal canal, contributing to poor healing.

INVESTIGATIONS
Diagnosis may be made by history and examination. Investigations are to exclude other conditions such as inflammatory bowel disease and rectal cancer.
Examination under anaesthesia to exclude other pathology if no response to treatment.

MANAGEMENT
Conservative: Ensure stools are soft and easily passed.
Medical: Topical GTN or diltiazem. These reduce spasm of the sphincter and increase local blood flow to encourage wound healing.
Surgery: Classically, a lateral internal sphincterotomy may be performed where a part of the internal sphincter is incompletely divided laterally to reduce spasm and therefore allow wound healing in the posterior midline. More recently, botulinum toxin (Botox) has been used to cause paralysis of part of the internal sphincter to achieve the same effect. Anal advancement flap in chronic fissures.

COMPLICATIONS
Chronic fissure and chronic pain.
Complications of surgery include faecal incontinence, bleeding recurrence.

PROGNOSIS
Recurrence is common, up to 50% of patients treated with topical nitrates and in less than 10% with lateral sphincterotomy.

Angiodysplasia

DEFINITION
GI mucosal vascular ectasias (dilatations) most commonly occurring in the colon.

AETIOLOGY
Exactly unknown but thought to be acquired as a degenerative process, possibly resulting from chronic, low-grade obstruction of submucosal veins.
Angiodysplasias often occur in the caecum and ascending colon, although the left colon can also be affected.

EPIDEMIOLOGY
Present in ~6% of those undergoing colonoscopy for variable indications and more common in the elderly (~25% in >60 years, most remaining asymptomatic).

HISTORY
Presents with bleeding PR, can be acute and rapid, characteristically intermittent with spontaneous cessation. Rebleeding is common.

EXAMINATION
Signs of shock if significant blood loss (hypotension, tachycardia). No characteristic signs on abdominal examination.

INVESTIGATIONS
Blood: FBC, U&Es, clotting, crossmatch (six units if significant bleed).
Endoscopy: Upper GI endoscopy should be carried out in cases of massive haemorrhage when source unknown. Once stable and can tolerate bowel preparation, colonoscopy.
Imaging: Angiography of superior or inferior mesenteric arteries shows vascular tufts in the capillary phase and early filling of dilated veins (>1 mL/minute blood loss required to visualise bleeding source). Radionucleotide scanning: ^{99m}Tc-labelled RBCs can detect bleeding of 0.5 mL/minute, but lacks spatial discrimination.

MANAGEMENT
Emergency: Assessment of haemodynamic status and resuscitation, O_2, IV access and fluids, blood transfusion if required. Correct any coagulopathy or give antifibrinolytics. With significant bleeds, invasive monitoring may be necessary (CVP monitoring and urinary catheter).
Endoscopic: May be treated by diathermy or photocoagulation during colonoscopy. On colonoscopy, the lesions are visible as small, raised or flat 'cherry-red' areas. Twenty-five per cent of cases are multiple.
Interventional radiology: Angiography and selective embolisation of bleeding vessels (can have serious complications, e.g. bowel ischaemia). Preferable to surgery as bleeding point may not be obvious at surgery.
Surgery: Need is dictated by rate and severity of blood loss and availability of interventional radiology. Following anterograde colon lavage by placement of a catheter in the appendix stump; on-table colonoscopy can be used to confirm the location of the bleeding and a segmental resection and primary anastomosis or a subtotal colectomy performed.

COMPLICATIONS
Haemorrhage, hypovolaemic shock, complications of investigations and treatment.

PROGNOSIS
Bleeding is usually self-limiting. Approximately 50% of those with bleeding episodes treated conservatively with observation and transfusion will continue to have episodes during the next few years.

Colon cancer

DEFINITION
Adenocarcinoma of the large bowel. Also see Rectal Cancers (page 98).

AETIOLOGY
Environmental and genetic factors have been implicated. A sequence from epithelial dysplasia to adenoma and then carcinoma is thought to occur involving accumulation of genetic changes, activation of oncogenes (e.g. APC, K-ras) and inactivation of tumour suppressor genes (e.g. p53, DCC). Please see **Associations/Risk Factors**

ASSOCIATIONS/RISK FACTORS
Colorectal polyps, previous colorectal cancer, inflammatory bowel disease (particularly long-standing ulcerative colitis). Genetic syndromes (familial adenomatous polyposis and Lynch syndrome) associated with ↑ risk (see Colonic Polyps).

EPIDEMIOLOGY
Third most common cancer and second cause of cancer death in the UK with ~37,500 cases/year. Average age at diagnosis 60–65 years. Rectal carcinomas male>female, colon carcinomas female>male.

HISTORY
Symptoms depend on the size and location of the tumour.
Patients may be asymptomatic and present with positive faecal occult blood tests via the NHS bowel cancer screening program.
Left-sided colon and rectum: Change in bowel habit, rectal bleeding or blood/mucus mixed in with stools. Rectal masses may also present as tenesmus (sensation of incomplete emptying after defecation).
Right-sided colon: Later presentation, with symptoms of anaemia, weight loss and non-specific malaise or, more rarely, lower abdominal pain.
Approximately 20% of tumours will present as an emergency with pain and distension due to large-bowel obstruction, haemorrhage or peritonitis due to perforation.

EXAMINATION
May be no signs.
Anaemia may be the only sign, particularly in right-sided lesions, abdominal mass, with metastatic disease, hepatomegaly, 'shifting dullness' of ascites.
Low-lying rectal tumours may be palpable on rectal examination.

PATHOLOGY/PATHOGENESIS
Sixty per cent rectum and sigmoid colon, 30% in the ascending colon and the remainder in the descending and transverse colon. Tumours can be annular, appearing as 'apple core' lesions (see Fig. 7) or form polypoid, exophytic masses. Staging systems include Dukes' (see Table below) and the TNM system (see Rectal Cancer, page 98).

INVESTIGATIONS
Blood: FBC (for anaemia), LFT, tumour markers (CEA to monitor treatment response or disease recurrence).
Stool: Occult or frank blood in stool (can be used as a screening test).
Endoscopy: Sigmoidoscopy, colonoscopy. Allows visualisation and biopsy. Polypectomy or endoscopic mucosal resection can be performed on isolated small carcinoma *in situ* lesions.
Imaging: Barium enema, CT scan, MRI, endorectal ultrasound, PET scanning. Please see **Pathology/Pathogenesis**.

MANAGEMENT
Screening: Reduces mortality by diagnosis and treatment of pre-malignant polyps and early disease.

Colon cancer (continued)

Surgery: Operation depends on site and stage, e.g.
- *Caecal tumours*: Right hemicolectomy.
- *Transverse colon tumours*: Extended right hemicolectomy.
- *Descending colon tumours*: Left hemicolectomy.
- *Sigmoid tumours*: Anterior resection.
- *High mid-rectal*: Anterior resection with total mesorectal excision.
- *Low rectal*: Abdominoperineal resection if unable to achieve clearance below tumour.
- *Emergency*: Depends on site and clinical presentation, examples: tumour resection and Hartmann's procedure, resection, primary anastomosis and defunctioning ileostomy.

Radiotherapy: May be given in a neoadjuvant setting to downstage rectal tumours prior to resection or as adjuvant therapy to reduce risk of local recurrence.

Chemotherapy: Used as adjuvant therapy or metastatic disease. Combination chemotherapy regimes with 5-fluorouracil are common (e.g. FOLFOX). In metastatic disease, bevacizumab (anti-vascular endothelial growth factor) or cetuximab (anti-epidermal growth factor receptor if no **K-ras** mutation) are used in combination with chemotherapy.

COMPLICATIONS
Bowel obstruction or perforation, fistula formation, recurrence, metastatic disease.

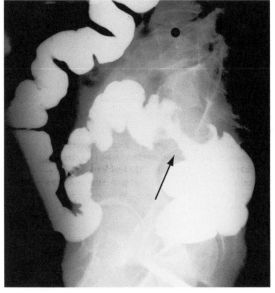

Figure 7 Barium enema study showing an 'apple-core' appearance indicative of a stenosing colonic carcinoma.

PROGNOSIS

Varies depending on stage. Those with defective mismatch repair have been shown to be associated with better outcome in resectable cases.

Dukes	Extent of spread	5-year survival
A	Confined to bowel wall	90–95%
B	Breached serosa but no lymph nodes involved	77%
C	Breached serosa with lymph nodes involved	48%
D*	Distant metastases (liver)	5–10%

*D stage is not part of the original Duke's staging.

Colonic polyps

DEFINITION

A growth or protruberence from the bowel wall that projects into the colonic lumen.

AETIOLOGY

Classified into non-neoplastic (hyperplastic, inflammatory pseudopolyps, hamartomatous) and neoplastic polyps, most of which are benign proliferations of mucosa and submucosa (adenomas), but clinically significant due to malignant potential (see Colon Cancer). Multiple polyp syndromes include the following:

Disorder	Features
Peutz–Jeghers syndrome	Diffuse GI polyposis with mucocutaneous pigmentation of lips and gums. Benign.
Familial polyposis coli	Multiple stomach, small and large bowel adenomas. Autosomal dominant APC gene. Pre-malignant.
Gardner's syndrome	Osteomas, soft tissue tumours, sebaceous cysts, congenital hypertrophy of RPE and multiple colonic adenomas. Pre-malignant.
Turcot's syndrome	Glioblastomas or medulloblastomas, with multiple colonic adenomas. Pre-malignant.
Cronkhite–Canada's syndrome	Alopecia, nail atrophy, pigmentation, watery diarrhoea, multiple colonic adenomas. Pre-malignant.

EPIDEMIOLOGY

Common. Prevalence is >50% in those >60 years.

HISTORY

Usually asymptomatic, occasionally cause bleeding, mucoid diarrhoea and anaemia or act as a lead point for intussusception.

EXAMINATION

Usually no findings on examination.
May be palpable on PR examination if low in rectum.

INVESTIGATIONS

Blood: FBC (anaemia).
Stool: Occult or frank blood in stool.
Endoscopy: Colonoscopy is gold standard investigation. For multiple polyposis syndromes, an upper GI endoscopy is necessary to look for upper GI polyps. Polyps removed need to be histologically examined to diagnose polyp type.

MANAGEMENT

Endoscopic treatment: Polypectomy, endoscopic mucosal resection. Transanal endoscopic microsurgery for large rectal polyps.
Surgical: Large polyps may have to be surgically resected. In multiple polyposis syndromes (particularly familial polyposis coli), early subtotal colectomy is recommended to reduce risk of malignancy.
Follow-up: Patients should be followed up with colonoscopy at intervals, depending on the type, size and number of polyps. Genetic screening of relatives may be necessary in multiple polyposis syndromes.

COMPLICATIONS

Malignant change with highest risk in villous adenomas and multiple polyposis syndromes.

PROGNOSIS

Good if detected and treated before any malignant change. The time for development of adenomas to cancer is about seven years.

Crohn's disease

DEFINITION
Chronic granulomatous transmural inflammatory bowel disease that can affect any part of the GI tract.

AETIOLOGY
Cause has not yet been elucidated, thought to involve an interplay between genetic and environmental factors.

ASSOCIATIONS/RISK FACTORS
- *Genetic:* NOD2 gene, HLA-B27 in those with ankylosing spondylitis
- *Environmental:* Smoking (4–6 times risk), refined sugar intake. Link to infectious agents (e.g. mycobacterium) proposed.

EPIDEMIOLOGY
Annual UK incidence is 5–8/100,000. Prevalence is 50–80/100,000. Affects any age but peak incidence is in young adults.

HISTORY
Crampy abdominal pain (due to transmural and peritoneal inflammation, fibrosis or obstruction of bowel), diarrhoea (may be bloody or steatorrhoea). Fever, malaise, weight loss. Symptoms of complications.

EXAMINATION
Weight loss, clubbing, signs of anaemia.
Aphthous ulceration of the mouth, perianal skin tags, fistulae and abscesses.
Signs of complications.

PATHOLOGY/PATHOGENESIS
Inflammation can occur anywhere along GI tract (40% involving the terminal ileum), 'skip' lesions with inflamed segments of bowel interspersed with normal segments. Mucosal oedema and ulceration with 'rose-thorn' fissures (cobblestone mucosa), fistulae, abscesses. Transmural chronic inflammation with infiltration of macrophages, lymphocytes and plasma cells. Granulomata with epithelioid giant cells may be seen in blood vessels or lymphatics.

INVESTIGATIONS
Blood: FBC ($\downarrow$ Hb, $\uparrow$ PLTs, $\uparrow$ WCC), U&Es, LFT ($\downarrow$ albumin), $\uparrow$ ESR, CRP ($\uparrow$ or may be normal), haematinics (to look for deficiency states), anti-*Saccharomyces cerevisiae* antibodies (ASCA).
Stool microscopy and culture.
Imaging: AXR: for evidence obstructions, toxic dilatation. Erect CXR: if risk of perforation. Small-bowel follow-through: may reveal fibrosis or strictures (string sign of Kantor), deep ulceration (rose-thorn), cobblestone mucosa (see Fig. 8). CT scanning, MRI for perianal disease.
Endoscopy (OGD, colonoscopy) and biopsy: May help to differentiate between ulcerative colitis and Crohn's disease, useful monitoring for malignancy and disease progression.

MANAGEMENT
Acute exacerbation: Fluid resuscitation, IV or oral corticosteroids, antibiotics, analgesia, high-dose 5-ASA analogues, e.g. mesalazine, sulphasalazine may induce a remission in Crohn's disease. DVT prophylaxis is important if unwell. Elemental diet may induce remission (more often used in children). Parenteral nutrition may be necessary.
Monitor: Temperature, pulse, respiratory rate, BP and markers of activity (ESR, CRP, platelets, stool frequency, Hb and albumin). Assess for complications. To measure progress, the Crohn's disease activity index can be used (score for number of stools,

Crohn's disease (continued)

abdominal pain, general wellbeing, symptoms related to findings, antidiarrhoeal medications, haematocrit and weight).

Long-term: Steroids for acute exacerbations, regular 5-ASA analogues to ↓ number of relapses in Crohn's colitis. For maintenance, steroid-sparing agents (e.g. azathioprine, risk of bone marrow suppression). The anti-TNF monoclonal antibody infliximab is used in severe or refractory cases, especially in fistulating disease.

Advice: Stop smoking, dietitian referral. Education and advice (e.g. from IBD nurse specialists).

Surgery: Indicated for failure of medical treatment, failure to thrive in children or the presence of complications. This does not prevent recurrence as disease can occur at another GI site.

COMPLICATIONS

Gastrointestinal: Haemorrhage, bowel strictures, perforation, fistulae (between bowel, skin, bladder, vagina), perianal fistulae and abscess, GI carcinoma (5% risk at 10 years), malabsorption, nutritional deficiencies.

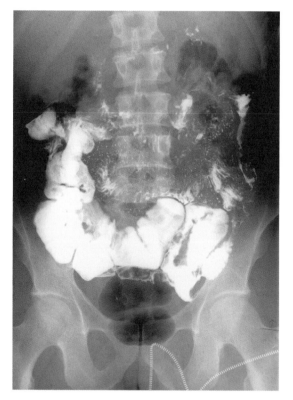

Figure 8 Barium enema demonstrating 'rose-thorn' and cobblestone appearances suggestive of Crohn's disease.

Extraintestinal: Uveitis, episcleritis, gallstones, kidney stones, arthropathy, sacroiliitis, ankylosing spondylitis, erythema nodosum and pyoderma gangrenosum, amyloidosis, thromboembolism.

PROGNOSIS

Chronic relapsing condition. Two-thirds will require surgery at some stage and two-thirds of these more than one surgical procedure. Increased risk of GI malignancy.

Diverticular disease

DEFINITION

Diverticulosis: The presence of diverticulae (Figs. 9,10), outpouchings of the colonic mucosa and submucosa through the muscular wall of the large bowel.

Diverticular disease: Diverticulosis associated with complications, e.g. haemorrhage, infection, fistulae.

Diverticulitis: Acute inflammation and infection of colonic diverticulae.

Hinchey's classification of acute diverticulitis: Ia: phlegmon, Ib and II: localised abscesses, III: perforation with purulent peritonitis or IV faecal peritonitis.

AETIOLOGY

A low-fibre diet leads to loss of stool bulk. Consequently, high colonic intraluminal pressures must be generated to propel the stool, leading to herniation of the mucosa and submucosa through the muscularis.

EPIDEMIOLOGY

Common, 60% of people living in industrialised countries will develop colonic diverticulae, rare <40 years. Right-sided diverticulae are more common in Asia.

HISTORY

Often asymptomatic (80–90%). Complications include PR bleeding, diverticulitis: typically, left iliac fossa or lower abdominal pain, fever. Diverticular fistulation into bladder: pneumaturia, faecaluria and recurrent UTI.

EXAMINATION

Diverticulitis: tender abdomen; signs of local or generalised peritonitis if perforation has occurred.

PATHOLOGY/PATHOGENESIS

Diverticulae are most common in the sigmoid and descending colon but can be right sided. Absent from the rectum. Diverticulae consist of herniated mucosa and submucosa through the muscularis, particularly at sites of nutrient artery penetration (see Fig. 9). Proposed

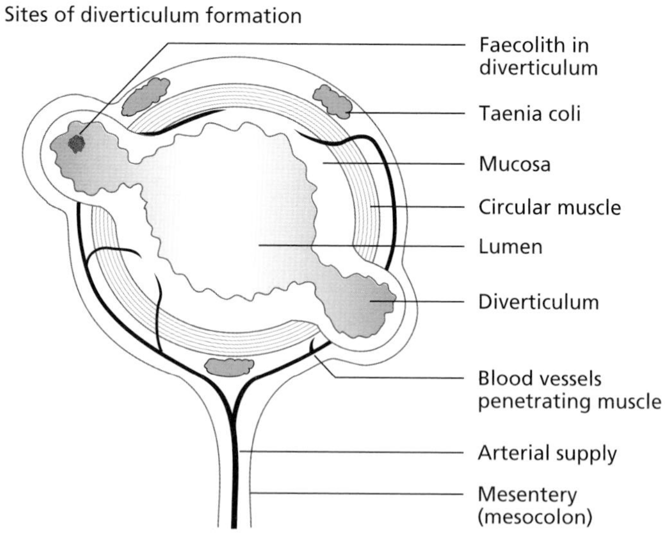

Sites of diverticulum formation

- Faecolith in diverticulum
- Taenia coli
- Mucosa
- Circular muscle
- Lumen
- Diverticulum
- Blood vessels penetrating muscle
- Arterial supply
- Mesentery (mesocolon)

Figure 9 Anatomy of colonic diverticulae.

diverticular obstruction by inspissated faeces can lead to bacterial overgrowth, toxin production and mucosal injury and diverticulitis, perforation, pericolic phlegmon, abscess, ulceration and fistulation or stricture formation.

INVESTIGATIONS

Blood: FBC, ↑ WCC and ↑ CRP in diverticulitis, check clotting and crossmatch if bleeding.

Barium enema (± air contrast): Demonstrates the presence of diverticulae with a sawtooth appearance of lumen, reflecting pseudo-hypertrophy of circular muscle (should not be performed in acute setting as there is a danger of perforation) (see Figs. 10a and 10b).

Flexible sigmoidoscopy and colonoscopy: Diverticulae can be seen and other pathology (e.g. polyps or tumour) can be excluded.

In an acute setting, CT scan for evidence of diverticular disease and complications.

MANAGEMENT

Asymptomatic: High-fibre diet (20–30 g/day). Probiotics and anti-inflammatories (mesalazine) are under investigation for preventing recurrent flares of diverticulitis.

GI bleed: PR bleeding is often managed conservatively with IV rehydration, blood transfusion if necessary. Angiography and embolisation or surgery if severe.

Diverticulitis: Treated by IV antibiotics and IV fluid rehydration and bowel rest. Localised collections or abscesses may be treated by radiologically sited drains.

Surgery: May be necessary with recurrent attacks or when complications develop, e.g. perforation and peritonitis. Surgical treatment can be by open or laparoscopic approaches. Open: Hartmann's procedure (resection and stoma) or one-stage resection and anastomosis (risk of leak) ± defunctioning stoma. More recently, laparoscopic drainage, peritoneal lavage and drain placement can be effective.

COMPLICATIONS

Diverticulitis, pericolic abscess, perforation, faecal peritonitis, colonic obstruction, fistula formation (bladder, small intestine, vagina), haemorrhage.

PROGNOSIS

Ten to 25 per cent of patients will have one or more episodes of diverticulitis. Of these, 30% will have a second episode.

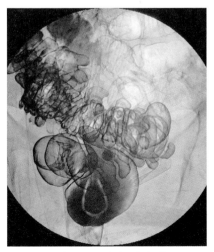

Figure 10 Air-contrast barium enema showing severe diverticular disease.

Gastrointestinal haemorrhage, lower

DEFINITION
Haemorrhage arising from the lower part of the gastrointestinal tract i.e. distal to the ligament of Treitz.

AETIOLOGY
Diverticular disease and angiodysplasia (account for 60–70%), colitis (inflammatory, ulcerative, infective, ischaemic, radiation), colonic polyps or carcinoma, haemorrhoids, anal fissures. More rarely, Meckel's diverticulum, solitary rectal ulcer, endometriosis, small bowel tumours, aorto-enteric fistula. Brisk upper GI bleeds can present with bleeding PR.

EPIDEMIOLOGY
Common, although less frequent than upper GI bleeds (account for 10–30% of GI bleeds). More common in older individuals.

HISTORY
Bloody diarrhoea or fresh bleeding implies a bleed distal to the caecum.
History suggestive of cause, e.g. inflammatory bowel disease.

EXAMINATION
Signs of iron deficiency anaemia (chronic).
Signs of shock, orthostatic or overt hypotension, tachycardia, hypovolaemia (acute).

INVESTIGATIONS
Blood: FBC, U&Es, clotting, LFT, crossmatching of blood in large bleeds. Faecal occult blood testing (guaiac) is used for screening of occult blood loss.

Endoscopy: Sigmoidoscopy/colonoscopy; unless rate of bleeding is slow, blood will obscure views. Once bleeding has settled, it can be used for diagnosis and treatment of colonic lesions. In brisk, significant bleeds, OGD to exclude upper GI cause.

Mesenteric angiography: Can localise site of bleeding (sensitivity ~60%) but rates must be >0.5 mL/minute and occurring at the time of contrast injection to demonstrate site. CT and MR angiography are becoming increasingly used.

Scintigraphy: Radiolabelled ^{99m}Tc-RBC scan can detect bleeding of 0.1–0.35 mL/minute, less accurate special localisation. Technetium scan: for ectopic gastric mucosa in Meckel's diverticulum.

Laparotomy and enteroscopy: Examination of whole colon and small bowel for lesions externally and internally via a endoscope passed through the bowel wall.

MANAGEMENT
Resuscitation: Adequate IV access, active resuscitation and correction of coagulopathies. NG tube and OGD investigate for upper GI source. Close monitoring in a HDU/ITU setting in cases of significant bleeds. Most will settle with conservative management.

Interventional radiology: Angiography for localisation and transcatheter embolisation of the bleeding vessel or vasopressin infusion.

Endoscopic: In stable patients, lower GI endoscopy may also treat source, e.g. laser photocoagulation of angiodysplasia.

Surgical: For severe or recurrent bleeding or if endoscopic or angiographic treatment is not feasible or has failed, subtotal colectomy may be required.

COMPLICATIONS
Anaemia, collapse and hypovolaemic shock.

PROGNOSIS
Depends on cause, most will cease spontaneously. The most common cause of life-threatening lower GI bleeding is diverticular disease; however, 90% of diverticular bleeding will settle with conservative management. If severe GI bleeds, aggressive resuscitation and early intervention improve outcome.

Haemorrhoids

DEFINITION
Anal vascular cushions (that contribute to anal closure) become enlarged and engorged with a tendency to protrude, bleed or prolapse into the anal canal.
Classified by location:
- Internal (arising from superior haemorrhoidal plexus and lie above the dentate line)
- External (from inferior haemorrhoidal plexus, below dentate line)

Classified by degree of prolapse:
- *First degree*: Haemorrhoids that do not prolapse.
- *Second degree*: Prolapse with defaecation, but reduce spontaneously.
- *Third degree*: Prolapse and require manual reduction.
- *Fourth degree*: Prolapsed and not reducible.

AETIOLOGY
Please see **Associations/Risk Factors** and **Pathology/Pathogenesis**

ASSOCIATIONS/RISK FACTORS
Constipation, prolonged straining, pregnancy, portal hypertension.

EPIDEMIOLOGY
Common (prevalence 4–5%). Peak age is 45–65 years. Predominantly a disease of the Westernised world.

HISTORY
Commonly asymptomatic.
Bleeding, usually bright red blood, on toilet paper or dripping into pan after passage of stool, can be on surface of stool but never mixed within. Alarm symptoms should be absent (weight loss, anaemia, change in bowel habit, passage of clotted, dark blood or mucus mixed with stool). Other symptoms are itching, anal lumps or prolapsing tissue. External haemorrhoids that have become thrombosed can cause severe pain.

EXAMINATION
First- or second-degree haemorrhoids are not usually apparent on external inspection, and uncomplicated haemorrhoids are impalpable and only seen on proctoscopy, where they are evident as red granular mucosal swellings bulging into view on straining and withdrawal of the proctoscope at 3, 7 and 11 o'clock. Differential diagnoses include anal tags, anal fissure, rectal prolapse, polyps or tumour.

PATHOLOGY/PATHOGENESIS
Excessive straining causes engorgement of anal cushions, together with shearing by hard stools resulting in disruption of tissue organisation, hypertrophy and fragmentation of muscle and elastin fibres and downward displacement, raised resting anal pressures and bleeding from pre-sinusoidal arterioles.

INVESTIGATIONS
Rigid or flexible sigmoidoscopy is usually important to exclude a rectal source of bleeding as haemorrhoids are common and may coexist with colorectal tumours.

MANAGEMENT
Conservative: Advice on a high-fibre diet, ↑ fluid intake, bulk laxatives. Topical creams are available that contain mild astringents combined with local anaesthetic; those with corticosteroids should only be used on a short-term basis.

Local therapy (for first or second degree): *Injection sclerotherapy:* 5% phenol in almond oil is injected above the dentate line (no sensory fibres) into the submucosa above a haemorrhoid, inducing inflammation and subsequent fibrosis resulting in mucosal fixation. *Banding:* Barron's bands are applied just proximal to the haemorrhoid-incorporating tissue that falls away after 2–3 days, leaving a small ulcer to heal by

Haemorrhoids (continued)

secondary intention. Higher cure rates but can be more painful. Other techniques include infrared coagulation, radio frequency ablation and heamorrhoidal artery ligation.

Surgical: Reserved for symptomatic third- or fourth-degree haemorrhoids. Milligan–Morgan open haemorrhoidectomy involves excision of haemorrhoidal cushions with preservation of skin/mucosal bridges between haemorrhoids to avoid stricturing. Stapled haemorrhoidectomy involves mucosectomy 2 cm proximal to the dentate line to 'hitch up' the prolapsing anal lining and disrupting the proximal blood flow (↓ pain and shorter convalescence in randomised control trials). Post-op, laxatives to avoid constipation, metronidazole.

COMPLICATIONS

Bleeding, prolapse, and thrombosis. From injection sclerotherapy: prostatitis, perineal sepsis, rarely impotence, retroperitoneal sepsis or hepatic abscesses. From haemorrhoidectomy: pain, bleeding, recurrence, more rarely incontinence due to sphincteric injury, anal stricture.

PROGNOSIS

Often a chronic problem, with recurrence of symptoms necessitating repeat local treatments. Surgery can provide long-term relief for severe symptoms.

Perianal abscess and fistula

DEFINITION

Perianal abscess: A pus collection in the perianal region.

Perianal fistula: An abnormal chronically infected tract communicating between the perianal skin and either the anal canal or rectum.

Abscess types: Classified according to location: submucous, subcutaneous, intersphincteric, ischiorectal and pelvirectal abscesses.

Fistula types: Park's classification as superficial, intersphincteric, transsphincteric, suprasphincteric or extrasphincteric, or alternatively as low anal (below puborectalis) or high anal (at or above puborectalis) and pelvirectal (involving levator ani) (see Fig. 11).

AETIOLOGY

Obstruction and stasis of anal crypt glands leads to superinfection that spreads to perianal tissues. Fistulae may develop once abscess discharges or has been evacuated. They are also a complication of Crohn's disease, where multiple perineal fistulae may develop (pepperpot perineum).

May be associated with diabetes or malignancy (rectal carcinoma).

EPIDEMIOLOGY

Common, peak incidence third to fourth decade. More common in men.

HISTORY

Constant throbbing pain in the perineum. With fistulae, intermittent discharge (mucus or blood stained) near the anal region.

EXAMINATION

Localised tender perianal swelling or a small skin opening with discharge near the anus corresponding to the opening of a fistula. On PR, an area of induration corresponding to

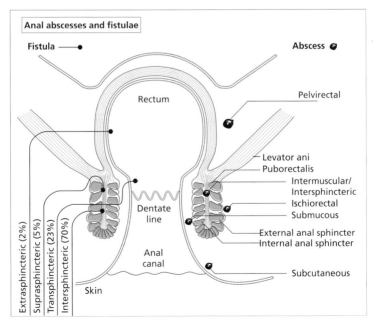

Figure 11 Perianal abscesses and fistulae.

Perianal abscess and fistula (continued)

the abscess or fistula tract may be felt. Not always possible due to pain or sphincter spasm. Examination under general anaesthesia may be warranted.

Goodsall's rule: Rule of thumb to correlate location of internal fistula opening based on location of external fistula opening. If external opening is anterior to the anal canal, the fistula runs radially and directly into the anal canal. If the external opening is posterior to the anal canal, the fistula tract follows a curved path, opening internally in the posterior midline (see Fig. 12).

INVESTIGATIONS

Blood: FBC, CRP, ESR, blood cultures if pyrexial.

For complex fistulae: MRI is extremely useful in allowing detailed study of the tracts. Allows for surgical planning ensuring complete excision.

Endoanal ultrasound: Also used, though less useful than MRI.

MANAGEMENT

Surgical: Requires surgical treatment under general anaesthesia.

Open drainage of abscess: Most common procedure is incision and drainage. A 'cruciate' incision is made over the abscess. Pus is removed and loculi broken down. The cavity is then irrigated and gently packed.

Laying open of fistula: A probe is used to gently explore the tract. Hydrogen peroxide or methylene blue can be injected into the external opening to demonstrate the internal opening.

Low fistulae: Treatment with a fistulotomy involves cutting down on and laying open the tract, curetting away granulation tissue and allowing healing by secondary intention. Extreme care must be taken to avoid damage to the anal sphincter.

High fistulae: For fistulae involving the upper half of the sphincter complex, where muscle division would cause incontinence, there are various surgical options. Seton – a non-absorbable suture that is threaded through the fistula tract – allows drainage of sepsis and gradually cuts through the sphincter in a manner that preserves continence. Advancement flap: The external part of the fistula is excised and the internal opening is closed by a mucosal advancement flap.

Fistula plug: A xenograft made from porcine intestinal submucosa is inserted into the tract to encourage closure. Fibrin glue – the fistula tract is obliterated with fibrin glue. Long-term results poor.

Antibiotics: Treatment of abscesses is surgical, and antibiotics are useful if there is surrounding cellulitis.

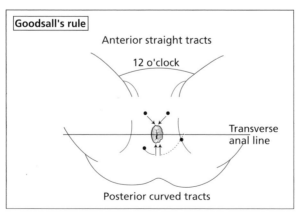

Figure 12 Goodsall's rule of perianal fistulae.

COMPLICATIONS

Recurrence, severe sepsis if untreated. Of fistula surgery: injury to the anal sphincter and incontinence.

PROGNOSIS

High recurrence rate without complete excision. Recurrence reported at between 0 and 63% with advancement flap for high fistulae.

Rectal cancer

DEFINITION
Cancer arising in the rectum. Accounts for approximately one-third of colorectal cancers.

AETIOLOGY
Genetic and environmental factors. Mutations lead to the cells escaping growth regulatory control, including activation of oncogenes and inactivation of tumour suppression genes. Adenomatous polyps can progress from severe dysplasia to neoplasia.

ASSOCIATIONS/RISK FACTORS
High-fat, low-fibre diet, presence of colorectal polyps, previous colorectal cancer, family history, inflammatory bowel disease (particularly long-standing ulcerative colitis). Familial syndromes (familial adenomatous polyposis, hereditary non-polyposis colorectal cancer).

EPIDEMIOLOGY
Around 14,000 new rectal cancer cases annually in the UK. Average age at diagnosis 60–65 years. Rectal carcinomas male>female.

HISTORY
Rectal bleeding or blood/mucus mixed in with stools is most common. Rectal masses may also present as a change in bowel habit or tenesmus (sensation of incomplete emptying after defecation). Patients may be asymptomatic and present with positive faecal occult blood tests via the NHS bowel cancer screening program.

EXAMINATION
Low-lying rectal tumours may be palpable on rectal examination, signs of anaemia, if obstructing lesions, abdominal distension. If metastatic disease, hepatomegaly, 'shifting dullness' of ascites. Rigid sigmoidoscopy should be performed.

PATHOLOGY/PATHOGENESIS
Most are adenocarcinomas (98%). Rarely, other tumour types include carcinoid, lymphoma, melanoma, sarcoma. Staging systems include the modified Dukes (see Colon Cancer, page 83) or the TNM staging system (see below).

INVESTIGATIONS
Blood: FBC (for anaemia), LFT, tumour markers (CEA).
Stool: Screening for faecal occult blood.
Endoscopy: Sigmoidoscopy, colonoscopy. Allows visualisation and biopsy. Polypectomy can also be done if isolated small carcinoma *in situ*.
Imaging: Staging by CT chest abdomen and pelvis, MRI rectum for local staging and planning treatment, endoanal ultrasound. PET scanning. Please see **Pathology/Pathogenesis**.

TNM Staging	
T1	Tumour invades submucosa
T2	Tumour invades muscularis propria
T3	Tumour invades into subserosa, pericolic or perirectal tissue
T4	Tumour invades other organs or through peritoneum
N0	No nodal metastases
N1	Metastases in 1–3 perirectal nodes
N2	Metastases in ≥4 perirectal nodes
N3	Nodal metastases along a vascular trunk
M0	No distant metastases
M1	Distant metastases

MANAGEMENT

Depends on stage and comorbid disease; management is planned by a multi-disciplinary team including surgeons, oncologists, gastroenterologists, pathologists and radiologists.

Transanal or endoscopic therapy: Pedunculated polyps or small early stage (in situ or T1) tumours may be treated by transanal excision or endoscopic mucosal resection. If any suspicion of nodal involvement, this should not be used.

Neoadjuvant chemotherapy and radiotherapy: Surgery alone has high local recurrence rate; this is improved by preoperative chemoradiotherapy (long course) or radiotherapy (short course). Benefits are down-staging, increased respectability and possible sphincter sparing.

Chemotherapy: Combination chemotherapy regimes with 5-fluorouracil are common (e.g. FOLFOX). In metastatic disease, bevacizumab (anti-vascular endothelial growth factor, anti-VEGF) and cetuximab (anti-EGFR, anti-epidermal growth factor receptor) can be used in combination with chemotherapy.

Surgery:

- Open or laparoscopic techniques. Anterior resection (for tumours of the middle and upper rectum, occasionally lower rectum if clear margins are achievable, usually 2 cm $\pm$ defunctioning stoma).
- Rectal surgery involves TME or total mesorectal excision, which reduces local recurrence rates.
- Abdominoperineal resection is used in cases where the anal sphincter cannot be preserved.
- In local recurrence or advanced tumours, a radical procedure called pelvic exenteration can be performed. This involves removal of the lower colon and rectum, along with lower ureters and bladder, internal reproductive organs, perineum, draining lymph nodes and pelvic peritoneum.
- Emergency: Hartmann's procedure or unresectable tumours may be defunctioned with proximal stoma.

COMPLICATIONS

Bowel obstruction or perforation, fistula formation, recurrence, metastatic disease. Complications associated with treatment. Surgery: anastomotic leak. Bleeding, ileus.

PROGNOSIS

5 year survival: Dukes A 80–90%; Dukes B 40–70%; Dukes C 12–40%; Dukes D 7–15%. With isolated liver metastases amenable to surgery, 5 year survival 25–40%.

Rectal prolapse

DEFINITION

The abnormal protrusion of rectal mucosa or full thickness rectal wall through the anus.

AETIOLOGY

Incomplete prolapse: When the prolapse only involves the mucosa, is seen in both children and adults and is associated with excessive straining, constipation and haemorrhoids.

Complete prolapse: Involves the entire rectal wall, occurring mainly in adults and associated with weak pelvic and anal musculature. Constipation, advanced age, chronic straining, sphincter paralysis, neurological conditions, e.g. multiple sclerosis, cystic fibrosis in children.

ASSOCIATIONS/RISK FACTORS

Please see **Aetilogy**

EPIDEMIOLOGY

Relatively common. Two peaks: in children <3 years (male = female) and the elderly (female : male is 6 : 1).

HISTORY

Protruding anal mass, may require digital replacement. Constipation, faecal incontinence, passing mucus or bleeding PR associated. May present as an emergency with irreducible or strangulated prolapse.

EXAMINATION

The prolapse may be seen on straining, with severity varying from protruding rectal mucosa to frank rectal prolapse (if >5 cm, invariably a complete prolapse). May be ulcerated or may show necrosis if vascular supply is compromised.

↓ anal sphincter tone.

INVESTIGATIONS

Imaging: Proctosigmoidoscopy, defaecating proctogram or barium enema.

Other: Anal sphincter manometry, pudendal nerve studies.

Sweat chloride test: In children, as ~10% will have cystic fibrosis.

MANAGEMENT

Conservative: Treatment for constipation with bulk laxatives. In children, a high-fibre diet and constipation treatment is usually sufficient.

Emergency: Acute prolapse may be manually reduced after adequate analgesia; there will be significant oedema and patients are often nursed, head down, with ice packs topically prior to attempted manual reduction; if the bowel is gangrenous, excision by rectosigmoidectomy.

Surgical:

Incomplete prolapse: Submucosal injection sclerotherapy with phenol-in-oil, mucosal banding or haemorrhoidectomy can be performed.

Complete prolapse: Operative repair using laparoscopic, abdominal or perineal approaches, e.g. Ripstein rectopexy: The rectum is mobilised and secured to the sacrum with non-absorbable sutures. Resection rectopexy can be performed; Delorme's procedure: excision of the rectal mucosa with plication of the underlying rectal muscle. Anal sphincter repair may be required in some cases. Altemeir's procedure: excision of prolapsed rectum and sigmoid colon from below and coloanal anastomosis.

COMPLICATIONS

Mucosal ulceration, rectal bleeding and incontinence. Rarely, strangulation and necrosis of prolapsed bowel.

PROGNOSIS

Spontaneous resolution usually occurs in children. Generally good in adults with appropriate treatment, although there is a 15% recurrence rate.

Toxic megacolon

DEFINITION
Severe colitis associated with segmental or total dilation of inflamed colon.

AETIOLOGY
Most commonly due to a severe flare of ulcerative colitis, but also may occur in Crohn's disease, pseudo-membranous colitis (*Clostridium difficile* infection) and other infective colitides.

EPIDEMIOLOGY
May occur in 3–10% of patients with ulcerative colitis, less common in Crohn's disease and generally rare in infective aetiologies.

HISTORY
The patient is systemically unwell, abdominal cramps and pain. Urgency and bloody diarrhoea.

EXAMINATION
Pyrexia, tachycardia, hypotension, dehydration. Tender distended abdomen, ↓ or loss of bowel sounds.

PATHOLOGY/PATHOGENESIS
Inflammation extends into the muscular layers of the bowel wall. There is neurogenic loss of motor tone and resulting distension of the colon and risk of perforation. Mucosal sloughing and tissue necrosis with muscle thinning is seen on histological examination. Colonic bacterial overgrowth leads to systemic toxicity from absorption through inflamed colonic mucosa.

INVESTIGATIONS
Blood: FBC (WCC raised dramatically), U&Es (↓ K^+), Alb (↓), high CRP.
Radiology: AXR or CT scan will show a dilated (>6 cm) colon. If >10 cm, high risk of perforation, and an erect CXR should be performed to detect air under the diaphragm, indicating perforation. Barium enema is contraindicated as it may cause perforation.

MANAGEMENT
Medical: The optimal management of severe colitis is multi-disciplinary with input of gastroenterologists, surgeons and intensive care. Aggressive fluid resuscitation and intravenous antibiotics ± steroids depending on aetiology. In ulcerative colitis, IV cyclosporine therapy can be used. Early and regular surgical review is important with clinical deterioration and progressive dilatation on serial abdominal radiographs despite medical therapy indications for surgery.
Surgical: A third of patients come to urgent surgery. Total colectomy with ileostomy is the appropriate surgical treatment in most cases.

COMPLICATIONS
Perforation and peritonitis. Systemic sepsis.

PROGNOSIS
High mortality (20–30%), especially if perforation occurs.

Ulcerative colitis

DEFINITION
Chronic relapsing and remitting inflammatory disease affecting the large bowel.

AETIOLOGY
Unknown. Hypotheses include genetic susceptibility (chromosomes 12, 16), immune response to bacterial or self-antigens, environmental factors, altered neutrophil function, abnormality in epithelial cell integrity.

Positive family history of IBD (~15%). Associated with ↑ serum pANCA, primary sclerosing cholangitis.

ASSOCIATIONS/RISK FACTORS
Please see **Aetiology**

EPIDEMIOLOGY
Prevalence: 1/1500 (in the developed world). Higher prevalence in Ashkenazi Jews, caucasians. Uncommon before the age of 10, peak onset age 20–40 years. Equal sex ratio up to age 40, then higher in males.

HISTORY
Bloody or mucous diarrhoea (stool frequency related to severity of disease). Tenesmus and urgency. Crampy abdominal pain before passing stool, weight loss, fever. Symptoms of extra-GI manifestations.

EXAMINATION
Signs of iron deficiency anaemia, dehydration. Clubbing. Abdominal tenderness, tachycardia. Blood, mucus and tenderness on PR examination. Signs of extra-GI manifestations.

INVESTIGATIONS
Blood: FBC (↓ Hb, ↑ WCC), ↑ ESR or CRP, ↓ albumin, crossmatch if severe blood loss, LFT.
Stool: Culture as infectious colitis is a differential diagnosis. Faecal calprotectin – marker for disease severity.
AXR: To rule out toxic megacolon (see Toxic Megacolon).
Flexible sigmoidoscopy or colonoscopy (and biopsy): Determines severity, histological confirmation, detection of dysplasia.
Barium enema: Mucosal ulceration with granular appearance and filling defects (pseudopolyps), featureless narrowed colon, loss of haustral pattern (lead-pipe or hosepipe appearance) (see Fig. 13). Colonoscopy and barium enema may be dangerous in acute exacerbations (risk of perforation).

MANAGEMENT
Markers of activity: ↓ Hb, ↓ Alb, ↑ ESR or CRP and diarrhoea frequency (<4 per day is mild, 4–6 per day is moderate, >6 per day is severe), bleeding, fever.
Acute exacerbation: IV rehydration, IV corticosteroids, antibiotics, bowel rest, parenteral feeding may be necessary, and DVT prophylaxis. Monitor fluid balance and vital signs closely. If toxic megacolon develops, low threshold for proctocolectomy and ileostomy as perforation has a mortality of 30%.
- *Mild disease*: Oral or rectal 5-aminosalicylic acid (5-ASA) derivatives, e.g. sulphasalazine and/or rectal steroids.
- *Moderate to severe disease*: Oral steroids and oral 5-ASA. Immunosuppression with azathioprine, cyclosporine, 6-mercaptopurine, infliximab (anti-TNF monoclonal antibody).
Advice: Patient education and support. Treatment of complications. Regular colonoscopic surveillance.
Surgical: Indicated for failure of medical treatment, presence of complications or prevention of colonic carcinoma. Proctocolectomy with ileostomy or an ileoanal pouch formation.

COMPLICATIONS

Gastrointestinal: Haemorrhage, toxic megacolon, perforation, colonic carcinoma (in those with extensive disease for >10 years), gallstones and PSC.

Extra-gastrointestinal manifestations (10–20%): Uveitis, renal calculi, arthropathy, sacroiliitis, ankylosing spondylitis, erythema nodosum, pyoderma gangrenosum, osteoporosis (from steroid treatment), amyloidosis.

PROGNOSIS

A relapsing and remitting condition, with normal life expectancy.

Poor prognostic factors (ABCDEF): Albumin (<30 g/L), blood PR, CRP raised, dilated loops of bowel, eight or more bowel movements per day, fever (>38 °C in first 24 hours).

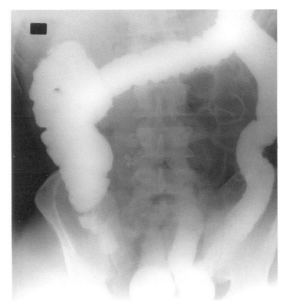

Figure 13 Barium enema showing featureless descending colon in ulcerative colitis.

Volvulus, colonic

DEFINITION
Rotation of a loop of bowel around the axis of its mesentery that results in bowel obstruction and potential ischaemia. The areas usually affected in adults are the sigmoid colon (65%) and caecum (30%).

AETIOLOGY
Anatomical factors, such as a long sigmoid mesentery, mobile caecum, chronic constipation and debility, age, very high residue diet, tumour, adhesions, Chagas' disease of the colon.

ASSOCIATIONS/RISK FACTORS
Please see **Aetiology**

EPIDEMIOLOGY
Causes ~5–10% of large bowel obstruction, more common in the elderly.

HISTORY
Abdominal pain and swelling, absolute constipation and later vomiting. There may be a history previous episodes with spontaneous resolution.

EXAMINATION
Signs of bowel obstruction with abdominal distension and tenderness. Tinkling or absent bowel sounds.

PATHOLOGY/PATHOGENESIS
Rotation of the segment of bowel results in partial or complete closed loop obstruction. With a 360° twist, the veins to the bowel are compressed and occluded, leading to circulatory impairment and, if not relieved, gangrene and perforation.

INVESTIGATIONS
AXR: Massively dilated loop of bowel, may have a 'coffee bean' shape. In caecal volvulus, the concavity of the coffee bean points to the right lower quadrant, and in sigmoid, to the left. May be associated with proximally dilated loops of bowel and distal collapse.
Water-soluble contrast enema: Demonstrates the site of obstruction; in sigmoid volvulus, there is a 'bird's beak' or 'ace of spades' deformity with spiral narrowing of the distal bowel at the site.
CT scan: Identifies rotation of mesentery and bowel as well as signs of bowel ischaemia.

MANAGEMENT
Resuscitation: Nil by mouth, IV fluids, NG tube if vomiting, IV antibiotics if signs of ischaemia/sepsis.
Endoscopic: Sigmoid volvulus may be managed by sigmoidoscopy and rectal tube insertion or flexible sigmoidoscopic decompression. In patients unfit for surgery with problematic recurrent sigmoid volvulus, sigmoid fixation by endoscopic placement of a percutaneous sigmoidostomy tube may be performed.
Surgical: If signs of peritonitis, bowel ischaemia or failure of conservative measures, laparotomy, untwisting, resection of dilated, gangrenous or ischaemic colon, with either a primary anastomosis and/or stoma formation. In the case of caecal volvulus, ileocaecal resection, right hemicolectomy or caecopexy is performed. Recurrent sigmoid volvulus may be treated by open or laparoscopic sigmoid colectomy.

COMPLICATIONS
Bowel obstruction, ischaemia and gangrene, toxaemia, bowel perforation, peritonitis.

PROGNOSIS
Conservative or endoscopic management of sigmoid volvulus is often effective, but recurrence is common. Overall mortality can be as high as 20%.

Cord compression and injury

DEFINITION
Injury to the spinal cord with neurological symptoms that depend on the site and extent of injury. Acute cord compression is an emergency.

AETIOLOGY
- direct contusion to the spinal cord from trauma;
- compression by bone/disc fragments or haematoma from trauma;
- compression from extrinsic lesions e.g.:
  ○ disc protrusion
  ○ tumours (primary bone, myeloma or secondary)
  ○ spinal abscesses (e.g. staphylococcus, TB)
  ○ spinal vascular malformations

EPIDEMIOLOGY
Common. Trauma occurs in all age groups. Malignancy and disc disease are more common in older ages.

HISTORY
History of injury or trauma or malignancy.
Pain, weakness, sensory loss.
Bowel or bladder function disturbance. Impotence.
Cauda-equina syndrome: Bilateral sciatica, saddle anaesthesia, urinary retention.
Brown–Séquard syndrome: Seen in hemisection of the spinal cord. Weakness of ipsilateral leg and numbness of contralateral leg.

EXAMINATION
Examine thoroughly for a motor and sensory level.
Acute cord trauma: Diaphragmatic breathing, reduced anal tone, hyporeflexia, priapism and spinal shock (↓ BP without tachycardia) are early hyperacute signs.
Cauda-equina syndrome: Flaccid paraparesis, urinary retention, reduced anal tone, saddle anaesthesia, impaired knee, ankle and bulbocavernous reflexes. May be asymmetrical.
Conus medullaris syndrome: Mixed flaccid and spastic paraparesis with urinary retention. Hypertonicity and hyperreflexia below the level of the lesion. Sensory disturbance tends to be in perianal distribution and symmetrical.
Brown–Séquard syndrome: Seen in hemisection of the spinal cord. Below the level of the lesion, there is ipsilateral spastic paralysis and loss of postural sense and contralateral loss of pain and thermal sense.
Distinguish cord compression from radiculopathies: Radiculopathies are caused by compression of the nerve root in the spinal canal or at the exit foramina. This causes LMN lesion only at that motor and sensory level but no UMN signs below the level.

Motor
C3–C5: Diaphragm
C5: Shoulder abduction
C6: Forearm flexion
C7: Forearm extension
C8: Wrist/finger flexion
T1: Finger abduction

L2: Hip flexion
L3: Knee extension
L4: Ankle dorsiflexion
L5: Big toe extension
S1: Ankle plantar flexion

Reflexes
C5–C6: Biceps reflex
C6: Brachioradialis (supinator) reflex
C7: Triceps reflex
Hoffmann's sign: UMN in upper limb

L1–L2: Cremaster reflex
L3–L4: Knee reflex
S1–S2: Ankle reflex
S2–S4: Anocutaneous reflex
S2–S4: Bulbocavernous reflex

Cord compression and injury (continued)

Sensory

C4: Supraclavicular fossa

C5: Clavicles

C6: Thumb

C7: Middle finger

C8: Little finger

T4: Nipples

T10: Umbilicus

T12: Hip girdle

L4: Medial malleolus

S1: Lateral malleolus

S2: Scrotum

S3–S5: Perianal region

INVESTIGATIONS

Trauma radiology: AP and lateral radiographs of cervical (also peg view), thoracic or lumbar spine. This is increasingly superseded by high-resolution CT scan of spine which allows reformatting for 3D visualisation.

Emergency MRI spine: To visualise soft tissue and cord. Cord signal change and canal stenosis are key features to identify (see Fig. 14)

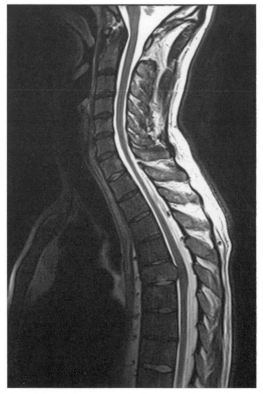

Figure 14 MRI showing thoracic cord compression from mass extending from the fourth thoracic veterbrae.

Blood: FBC, U&E, bone profile, Ca^{2+}, ESR, protein electrophoresis.
Urine: Bence Jones protein (indicative of multiple myeloma).

MANAGEMENT

Traumatic cord injury: Traumatic injuries should be managed according to ATLS guidelines. Use of high-dose steroids (methylprednisolone) in traumatic spinal cord injury is controversial, but the evidence from NASCIS trials favour motor benefit if given <8 hours in closed cord injury.

Cord compression: Following imaging, if a tumour is present, high-dose steroids (dexamethasone) should be given promptly to reduce cord compression. Tumours may also respond to emergency radiotherapy. Obtain neurosurgical advice.

Surgery: Necessary in a number of cases to relieve compression and/or remove cause of compression.

External surgical stabilisation: For example, by traction or halo device.

Internal surgical stabilisation: For example, by bone grafts or metal implants.

Surgical decompression: For example, laminectomy to relieve compression.

Discectomy or microdiscectomy: For disc prolapses.

Rehabilitation: Multi-disciplinary rehabilitation programme (preferably in specialist spinal unit) with physiotherapy and occupational therapy.

COMPLICATIONS

With severe injury, there is loss of spinal function below the level of the lesion.

Lesion above C4: Respiratory paralysis.

C4–T1: Quadriplegia.

Mid-thoracic: Paraplegia, autonomic dysreflexia, if above T6.

S1: Loss of sacral parasympathetic control over bladder and rectum.

Complications of immobility: Chest and urinary sepsis, pressure sores, DVT, long-term spasticity (with risk of deformity), heterotopic ossification.

PROGNOSIS

The American Spinal Injury Association (ASIA) Impairment Scale at 72 hours post-injury has prognostic value especially when converted to the Frankel grade (see: *www.asia-spinalinjury.org* for scoring sheet). There is some improvement in the longer term, depending on completeness of cord injury.

Extradural haemorrhage

DEFINITION

Bleeding and accumulation of blood into the extradural space.

AETIOLOGY

Head trauma causes a fracture (most commonly of the squamous temporal bone as this is the thinnest part of the cranial vault) which can rupture the middle meningeal artery. The arterial bleeding causes rapid accumulation of blood and strips the dura from the inner table of the skull. This results in raised ICP and compression of the underlying brain parenchyma.

EPIDEMIOLOGY

Annual incidence of 20/100,000 in the UK, 10% of severe head injuries. Most commonly seen in young adults. Uncommon in the elderly (subdural haemorrhages are more common in this age group).

HISTORY

Head injury with a temporary loss of consciousness, followed by a lucid interval, then development of progressive deterioration in conscious level.

EXAMINATION

Signs of scalp trauma or fracture.

Headache.

Deteriorating GCS.

Signs of raised ICP (e.g. dilated unresponsive pupil on the side of the injury).

Abnormal posturing (decorticate and decerebrate) and Cushing's sign (rising BP and bradycardia) are late signs.

INVESTIGATIONS

Urgent CT scan: Diagnostic and identifies location of haematoma. An arterial bleed produces a convex or lens-shaped haematoma. Signs of raised ICP include midline shift, compression of ventricles, obliteration of basal cisterns and sulcal effacement.

MANAGEMENT

Early management of head injuries: Follow ATLS guidelines to establish ABC and cervical spine control. Once stabilised, assessment is made of severity of head injury with an urgent CT scan.

Surgical: Urgent craniotomy and decompressive evacuation of the haematoma with diathermy or clipping of source of bleeding. An ICP monitor may be placed for post-op monitoring. Close observation and supportive care is required, often in an ITU setting.

COMPLICATIONS

Acutely; the greatest risk is cerebral herniation and death.

In the longer term, there may be associated post-traumatic brain injury, amnesia and cognitive impairment.

PROGNOSIS

Mortality rates relate to initial GCS and associated intracerebral injuries. If treated early, prognosis is good with underlying brain usually suffering limited injury.

Hydrocephalus

DEFINITION

Enlargement of the cerebral ventricular system (Fig. 15). Subdivisible into obstructive and non-obstructive (or communicating or non-communicating). *Hydrocephalus ex vacuo* is a term used to describe apparent enlargement of ventricles, but this is a compensatory change due to brain atrophy.

AETIOLOGY

Abnormal accumulation of CSF in the ventricles can be caused by:

1. impaired outflow of CSF from the ventricular system (obstructive):
   -lesions of the third ventricle, fourth ventricle, cerebral aqueduct,
   -posterior fossa lesions (e.g. tumour, blood) compressing the fourth ventricle,
   -cerebral aqueduct stenosis (Fig. 16);
2. impaired CSF resorption in the subarachnoid villi (non-obstructive):
   -tumours,
   -meningitis (typically tuberculosis),
   -normal pressure hydrocephalus (NPH), which is the idiopathic chronic ventricular enlargement. The long white matter tracts (corona radiata, anterior commissure) are damaged causing gait and cognitive decline.

EPIDEMIOLOGY

Bimodal age distribution. Congenital malformations and tumours in the young, tumours and strokes in the elderly.

HISTORY

Obstructive hydrocephalus: Acute drop in conscious level. Diplopia.
NPH: Chronic cognitive decline, falls, urinary incontinence.

EXAMINATION

Obstructive hydrocephalus: Impaired GCS, papilloedema, VI nerve palsy ('false localising sign' of increased ICP). In neonates, the head circumference may enlarge, and 'sunset sign' (downward conjugate deviation of eyes).
NPH: Cognitive impairment. Gait apraxia (shuffling). Hyperreflexia.

INVESTIGATIONS

CT head: First-line investigation to detect hydrocephalus. May also detect the cause (e.g. tumour in the brainstem).
Lumbar puncture: This is contraindicated in obstructive hydrocephalus as it can cause tonsillar herniation and death. May be necessary in normal pressure hydrocephalus as a therapeutic trial.

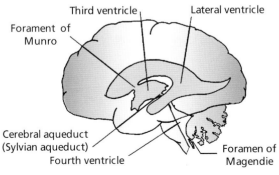

Figure 15 CSF ventricular drainage system.

Hydrocephalus (continued)

CSF: Obtained from ventricular drains or lumbar puncture may indicate an underlying pathology (e.g. tuberculosis). Check for MC&S, protein, glucose (CSF and plasma).

MANAGEMENT

Emergency: Airway, breathing and circulation. If GCS is impaired, protect and secure airway. Treat seizures. Obtain CT and liaise with neurosurgery urgently.

External ventricular drain: Insertion of a catheter into the lateral ventricle to bypass any obstruction.

Ventriculoperitoneal shunting: Implantation of a ventricular catheter into one or both lateral ventricles and connecting it to a subcutaneous drain which leads to the peritoneal cavity. Carries risk of shunt infection, block or malfunction (especially as some are electronic).

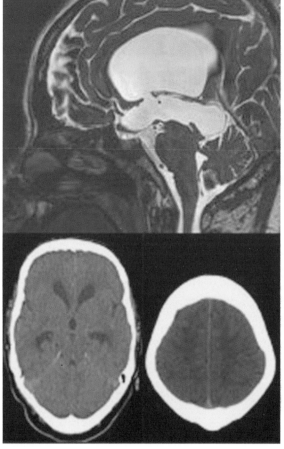

Figure 16 (Top) Lateral and third ventricle dilation due to central aqueduct stenosis; (bottom-left) enlarged temporal horns of the lateral ventricle; (bottom right) paucity of cerebral sulci indicative of raised ICP.

Lumboperitoneal shunting: Alternative procedure that may be suitable for communicating hydrocephalus.

Advanced neurosurgery: Endoscopic ventriculostomy and aqueductoplasty are other options used to bypass blockages or maintain patency for CSF flow.

COMPLICATIONS
Cerebral herniation, coning, death.

PROGNOSIS
Obstructive hydrocephalus is often fatal if untreated. Cognitive and gait decline in NPH can improve with shunting.

Intracerebral haemorrhage

DEFINITION
Haemorrhage within the brain parenchyma with formation of a focal haematoma.

AETIOLOGY
Hypertension and trauma are the most common causes. Other causes include arteriovenous malformation, intracerebral aneurysms, cavernous haemangiomas, tumours, bleeding into a previously infarcted region and drug abuse (e.g. amphetamine, cocaine).
May progress outwards onto the surface of the brain (becoming a subarachnoid haemorrhage) or inwards into the ventricular system (intraventricular haemorrhage).

EPIDEMIOLOGY
Fifteen per cent of strokes. Incidence is 15–300/100,000. Peak incidence in older age groups.

HISTORY
Sudden development of stroke syndrome, symptoms depending on the site of haemorrhage (e.g. contralateral weakness, speech disturbance if in dominant hemisphere).
Deteriorating level of consciousness.
Headache and vomiting.

EXAMINATION
Signs of stroke syndrome: Hemiparesis, sensory loss, cranial nerve lesions, cerebellar ataxia, loss of higher cognitive functions.
Signs of ↑ ICP: ↓ GCS, ↑ BP, bradycardia. Unequal pupils may indicate impending herniation.

INVESTIGATIONS
CT brain: Indicated for all strokes to distinguish ischaemic from haemorrhagic stroke. Features of severity include signs of raised ICP, midline shift and hydrocephalus.
MRI brain: Gradient-echo sequence has high sensitivity for haemosiderin and is useful for identifying areas of microhaemorrhage.
Cerebral angiography: May be indicated if suspicion of an underlying vascular malformation.

MANAGEMENT
Emergency: Attention to ABC; intubation and ventilation may be necessary with GCS. Supportive care with resuscitation and correction of coagulation and electrolyte abnormalities.
Surgery: Craniotomy for evacuation of haematoma should be reserved for large (>3 cm) cerebellar haemorrhages, or those with large lobar haemorrhages, substantial mass effect, and rapidly deteriorating condition as STICH-1 trial shows no significant benefit from early neurosurgery.
Medical: *ICP monitoring*: Monitoring (e.g. insertion of pressure monitoring bolt) and treatment of ↑ ICP (e.g. external ventricular drain in hydrocephalus, upright bed positioning, hyperventilation).
Blood-pressure control: Precipitous reduction of BP carries risk of causing watershed infarction. Standard guidelines recommend target systolic BP <180 mmHg, although the INTERACT trial has shown that a target systolic BP <140 mmHg is associated with reduced haematoma growth and no increased risk of adverse events.
Supportive: Nutritional support (NG feeding), care of pressure points, speech and language therapy, rehabilitation.
Newer agents: Factor VII decreases hematoma expansion, but there was no effect on outcome (FAST trial).

COMPLICATIONS
↑ ICP, hydrocephalus (especially in posterior fossa haemorrhage) herniation, neurological deficits.

PROGNOSIS
High mortality, with GCS score on admission and size of haematoma being strong predictors of prognosis.

Subarachnoid haemorrhage

DEFINITION
Haemorrhage into the subarachnoid space, the CSF-containing space between the arachnoid mater that lines the internal surface of the dura and the pia mater that covers the brain and the spinal cord.

AETIOLOGY
Eighty-five per cent rupture of a saccular (berry) aneurysm, 5% AVMs.
Other causes: trauma, perimesencephalic haemorrhage, mycotic aneurysms, drug abuse (e.g. cocaine).

EPIDEMIOLOGY
Annual incidence ~10/100,000. Peak age in the fifties.

HISTORY
Sudden onset severe headache, classically described 'as if hit at the back of the head'. Associated nausea, vomiting, neck stiffness, photophobia.
Confusion, collapse or ↓ level of consciousness.

EXAMINATION
Meningism: Neck stiffness, Kernig's sign (resistance or pain on knee extension when hip is flexed) due to irritation of the meninges by blood.
Glasgow Coma Scale: Assess and regularly monitor for deterioration.
The Glasgow Coma Scale (GCS) is made up of three components; the minimal score is 3, and the maximal score is 15.

Eye opening	Verbal response	Motor response
Spontaneously (4)	Oriented (5)	Obeying commands (6)
To speech (3)	Confused (4)	Localising pain (5)
To pain (2)	Inappropriate (3)	Flexion to pain (4)
None (1)	Incomprehensible (2)	Abnormal flexion to pain (3)
	None (1)	Extending to pain (2)
		None (1)

Signs of ↑ ICP: Papilloedema, IVth or IIIrd cranial nerve palsy (the latter may also be due to pressure from a posterior communicating artery aneurysm).
Fundoscopy: Subhyaloid haemorrhage (between retina and vitreous membrane).
Focal neurological signs: Often due to ischaemia from vasospasm and reduced brain perfusion.

PATHOLOGY/PATHOGENESIS
Abnormal localised dilatation of a blood vessel, usually seen at the sites of bifurcation of arteries in the circle of Willis where there is believed to be a congenital or acquired weakness in the vessel wall. Saccular aneurysms are associated with polycystic kidney disease, Marfan's syndrome, pseudoxanthoma elasticum and Ehlers–Danlos syndrome. Twenty per cent have multiple aneurysms.

INVESTIGATIONS
Blood: FBC, U&Es, ESR, CRP, clotting, G&S.
CT scan: Blood is seen as hyperdense areas in the subarachnoid space, commonly in the basal cisterns or Sylvian fissure. There may be associated hydrocephalus (see Fig. 17).
Angiography (MRI, CT or intra-arterial four-vessel): To detect the site of bleeding if the patient is a candidate for surgery or endovascular treatment.
Lumbar puncture: ↑ Opening pressure, ↑ RBC, low WCC, xanthochromia (straw-coloured CSF) due to breakdown of Hb, confirmed by spectrophotometry of CSF supernatant after centrifugation.

MANAGEMENT

Acute: Maintain ABC with IV fluids to maintain cerebral perfusion (use 0.9% saline – avoid dextrose as it may worsen hyponatraemia and ↑ cerebral oedema), bed rest, analgesics (paracetamol or codeine) and obtain urgent neurosurgical review. Nimodipine should be given 4 hourly to prevent vasospasm.

Interventional neuroradiology: Coiling (usually with platinum) of aneurysm. Outcome is similar if not superior to neurosurgery based on the ISAT trial.

Surgical: Clipping or wrapping of aneurysm may be necessary if aneurysm is not amenable to neuroradiological intervention.

COMPLICATIONS

Hydrocephalus due to blood obstructing CSF flow or resorption through the arachnoid villi (25%).

Cerebral vasospasm (occurring about 24–72 hours after haemorrhage).

Hyponatraemia (may be due to SIADH or cerebral salt-wasting syndrome).

Major neurological deficits depending on the site of haemorrhage.

PROGNOSIS

High mortality (>30% in the first few days). Those with a lower GCS or neurological deficit on presentation have a worse prognosis. Significant risk of a severe rebleed in the first 2 months without treatment. Lower mortality in cases of perimesencephalic subarachnoid haemorrhage than aneurysmal bleeds.

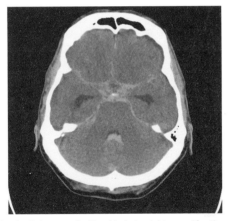

Figure 17 CT scan showing high attenuation (blood) in the basal cisterns and fourth ventricle and secondary hydrocephalus.

Subdural haemorrhage

DEFINITION

A subdural haematoma (SDH) is a collection of blood that develops between the surface of the brain and the dura mater.

Acute: Within 72 hours.

Subacute: Three to 20 days.

Chronic: After 3 weeks.

AETIOLOGY

Trauma causing rapid acceleration and deceleration of the brain results in shearing forces which tear veins ('bridging veins') that travel from the dura to the cortex. Bleeding occurs between the dura and arachnoid membranes.

In children, non-accidental injury should always be considered.

EPIDEMIOLOGY

Acute: Tend to occur in younger patients/associated with major trauma (5–25% of cases of severe head injury). More common than extradural haemorrhage.

Chronic: More common in the elderly, studies report incidence of 1–5/100,000.

HISTORY

Acute: History of trauma with head injury, patient has ↓ conscious level.

Subacute: Worsening headaches 7–14 days after injury, altered mental status.

Chronic: Can present with headache, confusion, cognitive impairment, psychiatric symptoms, gait deterioration, focal weakness, seizures.

There may not be a history of fall or trauma; hence have low index of suspicion especially in the elderly and alcoholics.

EXAMINATION

Acute: ↓ GCS. With large haematomas resulting in midline shift, an ipsilateral fixed dilated pupil may be seen (compression of the ipsilateral IIIrd nerve parasympathetic fibres), pressure on brainstem: ↓ consciousness, bradycardia.

Chronic: Neurological examination may be normal; there may be focal neurological signs (IIIrd or VIth nerve dysfunction, papilloedema, hemiparesis or reflex asymmetry).

INVESTIGATIONS

CT head: Crescent- or sickle-shaped mass (see Fig. 18), concave over brain surface (an extradural is lentiform in shape), CT appearance changes with time. Acute subdurals are hyperdense, becoming isodense over 1–3 weeks (such that presence may be inferred from signs such as effacement of sulci, midline shift, ventricular compression and obliteration of basal cisterns), and chronic subdurals are hypodense (approaching that of CSF).

MRI brain: Has higher sensitivity especially for isodense or small SDHs.

MANAGEMENT

Acute: ATLS protocol with priorities of cervical spine control and ABC. With a head injury, there is significant risk of cervical spine injury. Disability: GCS, pupillary reactivity. If signs of raised ICP, elevate the head and consider osmotic diuresis with mannitol and/or hyperventilation. Once stabilised, obtain CT head.

Conservative: Especially if small and minimal midline shift (SDH <10-mm thickness, and midline shift <5 mm).

Surgical: Prompt Burr hole or craniotomy and evacuation for symptomatic subdurals >10 mm, with >5-mm midline shift (better outcome if within 4 hours). ICP monitoring devices may be placed.

Chronic: If symptomatic or there is mass effect on imaging, surgical treatment with Burr hole or craniotomy and drainage (a drain may be left in for 24–72 hours). Asymptomatic SDH without significant mass effect is best managed conservatively with serial imaging to monitor for spontaneous resorption. Haematomas that have not fully liquefied may require craniotomy with membranectomy.

Children: Younger children may be treated by percutaneous aspiration via an open fontanelle or if this fails, placement of a subdural to peritoneal shunt.

COMPLICATIONS

Raised ICP, cerebral oedema predisposing to secondary ischaemic brain damage, mass effect (transtentorial or uncal herniation).

Post-op: Seizures are relatively common, recurrence (up to 33% for SDH), intracerebral haemorrhage, subdural empyema, brain abscess or meningitis, tension pneumocephalus.

PROGNOSIS

Acute: Underlying brain injury is the most important factor on outcome.

Chronic: Generally have a better outcome than acute SDHs, reflecting lower incidence of underlying brain injury, with good outcomes in three-fourths of those treated by surgery.

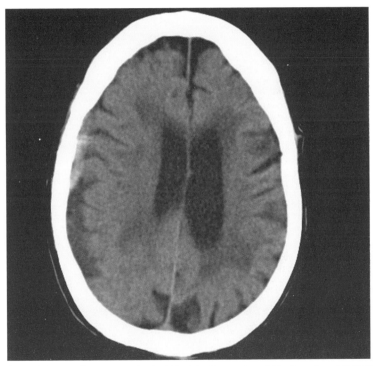

Figure 18 CT scan of an acute on chronic right subdural haemorrhage (high-attenuation white signal indicates fresh blood; lower attenuation indicates more mature blood).

Cataracts

DEFINITION
Opacification of the lens of the eye.

AETIOLOGY
Majority of cases are idiopathic age related ('senile cataracts').
    Numerous secondary causes include the following:
Local: Previous eye trauma, uveitis, intraocular tumours.
Systemic: Diabetes, metabolic disorders (galactosaemia, hypocalcaemia, Wilson's disease),
    skin disease (atopic dermatitis, scleroderma), drugs (steroids), X-ray and UV radiation,
    myotonic dystrophy, genetic syndromes (Down's).
Congenital: Congenital rubella syndrome.

EPIDEMIOLOGY
Major cause of treatable blindness worldwide. Thirty per cent of >65-year-olds have visually
impairing cataracts in one or both eyes, which increase with age.

HISTORY
Gradual onset painless loss of vision.
Glare from bright lights, vision may worsen in bright light (especially with central lens opacity).
Some may experience monocular diplopia and see haloes around lights.
Some may notice that they can read without glasses (nuclear sclerotic cataract may ↑ lens
    converging power).
In infants, there may be amblyopia or nystagmus.

EXAMINATION
Loss of red reflex and hazy lens appearance. Reduced visual acuity.

INVESTIGATIONS
Biometry: Required to assess appropriate intraocular lens (IOL) implant.
Others unnecessary unless occurring at an early age or associated with systemic disease.

MANAGEMENT
Congenital cataracts must be treated urgently to avoid amblyopia.
The decision for surgery depends on the effect of the cataracts on the patient's vision and life.
Surgical: Phacoemulsification (using ultrasound probe) followed by aspiration of lens material
    and insertion of intraocular lens implant is curative. Specific complications include posterior
    capsule opacification, vitreous humour loss, and endophthalmitis. Usually done under local
    anaesthesia as day surgery. Post-op care should include steroid drops (for inflammation),
    antibiotic drops (infection prophylaxis), avoidance of strenuous exercise and ocular trauma.

COMPLICATIONS
None, other than reduced quality of life from reduced visual acuity.

PROGNOSIS
Good with treatment for age-related cataracts.

Fracture, neck of femur

DEFINITION

Break in the continuity of cortical bone of the femur at or above the lesser trochanter. Fractures are classified into two categories:

- *Intracapsular*: Occur proximal to the point where the hip joint capsule attaches to the femur; includes subcapital, transcervical and basicervical.
- *Extracapsular*: Trochanteric (see Figs. 19a and 19b) or subtrochanteric.

AETIOLOGY

Osteoporosis and ↑ prevalence of falls in the elderly; other risk factors are current smoking, ↓ BMI (<18.5), previous low trauma fracture after 50 years of age, maternal history of hip fracture, hyperparathyroidism and Paget's disease.

Anatomy: As the principal blood supply to the femoral head is via retinacular vessels that travel back along the capsule, intracapsular fractures can interrupt supply and result in avascular necrosis.

EPIDEMIOLOGY

Common in the elderly, with lifetime risk of 18% in women, 6% in males. Prevalence 3/100 (65–74 years), 12/100 (>85 years).

HISTORY

History of fall may be minor, resulting in pain and restriction of movement in the hip area.

EXAMINATION

The affected leg is shortened, adducted and externally rotated, with pain in the hip.

INVESTIGATIONS

Blood: FBC, U&Es, clotting, G&S.

Imaging: Plain radiographs of AP and lateral views of the hip. If there is doubt regarding diagnosis, MRI, bone scan or repeat plain radiographs after a delay of 24–48 hours should be performed. CXR if elderly and surgery required.

MANAGEMENT

Prevention: Risk assessment and interventions aimed at reducing risk of falls.

Medical: Calcium, vitamin D, HRT, selective oestrogen receptor modulators, bisphosphonates, calcitonin, fluoride and thiazides have been used for primary or secondary prevention.

Immediate: Resuscitation, correction of fluid and electrolyte imbalance, analgesia and attention to pressure areas. Patients should be operated on within 24 hours, as this reduces the risk of thrombotic complications and pressure damage.

Undisplaced intracapsular fractures: Internal fixation allows early mobilisation and reduces risk of fractures becoming displaced; in the very elderly, hemiarthroplasty may be considered.

Displaced intracapsular fractures: Open reduction and internal fixation (younger, more active patients), hemiarthroplasty or total hip replacement (may be appropriate in patients with pre-existing joint disease, good activity levels and a reasonable life expectancy).

Extracapsular fractures: Should be treated surgically unless medical contraindication by reduction and internal fixation using extramedullary (e.g. sliding screw and plate) or intramedullary (e.g. Gamma nail implants).

All patients should receive antibiotic prophylaxis at induction and DVT prophylaxis.

COMPLICATIONS

Early: Pain, immobility, infections, DVT (asymptomatic up to 45%, symptomatic up to 11%) and PE (3–13%), pressure sores (20%), pulmonary complications (ARDS, fat embolism, pneumonia).

Late: Avascular necrosis of the femoral head, non-union and implant failure.

Fracture, neck of femur (continued)

PROGNOSIS

In the elderly mortality after hip fracture is high, 30% at 1 year, with 25% requiring a higher level of long-term care.

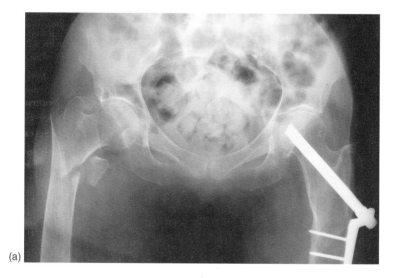

(a)

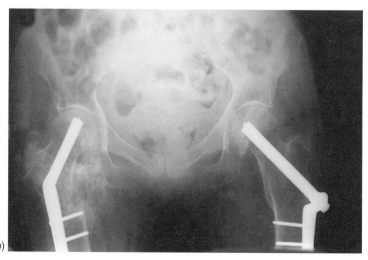

(b)

Figure 19 (a) A right trochanteric (extracapsular) fracture. (b) Same patient after reduction and internal fixation with a dynamic hip screw. The patient has had a previous fixation on the left side.

Septic arthritis

DEFINITION

Intra-articular joint infection.

AETIOLOGY

Bacteria enter the joint either directly, e.g. penetrating wound, by haematogenous spread from adjacent osteomyelitis or by a contaminated prosthesis. Bacteria in the joint incite an inflammatory response. Activation of neutrophils and macrophages results in release of proteolytic enzymes, which, together with bacterial toxins, cause damage to the articular cartilage. ↑ Permeability and fluid secretion result in a joint effusion. During recovery, healing of the raw articular surfaces may result in fibrosis and bony ankylosis.

The most common causative organisms in those <3 years are *Staphylococcus aureus*, *Haemophilus influenzae* or coliforms, and *S. aureus* and *Neisseria gonorrhoeae* in adults.

ASSOCIATIONS/RISK FACTORS

Diabetes, IV drug abuse, those immunocompromised or with chronic joint disease (e.g. rheumatoid arthritis) are at ↑ risk of septic arthritis.

EPIDEMIOLOGY

Incidence ~6/100,000, 50% of cases in children <3 years.

HISTORY

Pain in a joint or limb, malaise, fever.

Commonly affects a single large joint; e.g. the hip in infants and children, present with a limp and refusing to bear weight. The knee is often affected in older children and adults, although it may affect any joint.

EXAMINATION

A red swollen joint; if a hip, the leg is held flexed and slightly externally rotated (slackens ligaments and reduces joint pressure).

Diffuse joint tenderness with severe reduction in range of movement due to pain.

If gonococcal arthritis, there may be associated skin pustules near the joint.

INVESTIGATIONS

Blood: FBC, blood cultures, ESR, CRP.

Joint aspiration and microscopy, culture and sensitivity: Aspirate usually turbid with multiple neutrophils, culture to identify causative organism.

Joint radiograph: Shows ↑ joint space, soft tissue swelling and in late cases, subchondral bone destruction.

Bone scan: ↑ uptake is seen in joint region.

USS: To identify a joint effusion, may guide aspiration.

MANAGEMENT

Surgical: In most cases, surgical washout of the joint should be carried out to remove pus and infected material. May be performed by arthroscopy or open procedure (arthrotomy). Sepsis in a prosthetic joint requires removal of the prosthesis before full eradication of infection is possible.

Medical: Antibiotics initially IV for 1–2 weeks followed by oral for an additional 4–6 weeks. Analgesics should be given and the joint should be splinted for pain reduction. Physiotherapy is provided to prevent fibrosis and maintain joint mobility.

COMPLICATIONS

Joint subluxation or dislocation, avascular necrosis of epiphysis, growth disturbance, ankylosis, joint destruction or secondary osteoarthritis.

PROGNOSIS

Outcomes are dependent on the virulence of the organism, duration of infection prior to diagnosis, the pre-morbid condition of the patient and the joint affected; e.g. knees have better outcomes than ankles. With early appropriate treatment, prognosis is usually good.

Basal cell carcinoma (skin)

DEFINITION

Commonest form of skin malignancy; also known as a 'rodent ulcer'.

AETIOLOGY

Prolonged sun exposure or UV radiation. Associated with abnormalities of the *patched/ hedgehog* intracellular signalling cascade, as seen in Gorlin's syndrome (naevoid basal cell carcinoma syndrome). Other risk factors include photosensitising pitch, tar and arsenic.

EPIDEMIOLOGY

Common in those with fair skin and areas of high sunlight exposure, common in the elderly, rare before the age of 40 years. Lifetime risk in Caucasians is 1:3.

HISTORY

A chronic, slowly progressive skin lesion usually on the face but also on the scalp, ears or trunk.

EXAMINATION

Nodulo-ulcerative (most common): Small glistening translucent skin over a coloured papule that slowly enlarges (early) or a central ulcer ('rodent ulcer') with raised pearly edges. Fine telangiectatic vessels often run over the tumour surface. Cystic change may be seen in larger, more protuberant lesions.

Morphoeic: Expanding, yellow/white waxy plaque with an ill-defined edge (more aggressive).

Superficial: Most often on trunk, multiple pink/brown scaly plaques with a fine 'whipcord' edge expanding slowly; can grow to more than 10 cm in diameter.

Pigmented: Specks of brown or black pigment may be present in any type of basal cell carcinoma.

PATHOLOGY/PATHOGENESIS

Small dark blue staining basal cells growing in well-defined aggregates invading the dermis with the outer layer of cells arranged in palisades. Numerous mitotic and apoptotic bodies are seen. Growth rate is usually slow but steady and insidious. It does not metastasise, but has the potential to invade and destroy local tissues.

INVESTIGATIONS

Biopsy is rarely necessary (diagnosis is based mainly on clinical suspicion).

MANAGEMENT

Cryotherapy, curettage, cauterisation and photodynamic therapy are used for small superficial lesions.

Surgical: Excision with a 0.5 cm margin of surrounding normal skin for discrete nodular or cystic nodules; Mohs' micrographic surgery, which includes careful review of tissue excised under frozen section, is the treatment of choice for large tumours (1 cm diameter) and lesions near the eyes, nose and ears. Excision and skin flap coverage may be necessary.

Radiotherapy: Useful in basal cell carcinomas involving structures that are difficult to surgically reconstruct (e.g. eyelids, tearducts). Repeated treatments may be necessary, there is risk of side-effects such as radiation dermatitis, ulceration and depilation.

COMPLICATIONS

The tumour has a slow but relentless course. Can become disfiguring on the face. Has the potential to invade, lead to loss of vision in the orbital region.

PROGNOSIS

Good with appropriate treatment. If left, may continue to grow, invade and ulcerate. Regular follow-up is necessary to detect local recurrence or other lesions.

Burns

DEFINITION
Tissue damage that occurs by thermal, electrical or chemical injury.

AETIOLOGY
Contact with fire, hot object, liquids, electricity, UV light and irradiation, or chemicals.

EPIDEMIOLOGY
Common, >12,000 admissions in England and Wales annually.

HISTORY
Circumstances of burn, note time, temperature and length of contact with agent. Consider risk of inhalation of smoke and toxic gas poisoning (carbon monoxide). Consider non-accidental injury in children and vulnerable adults.

EXAMINATION
Look for signs of inhalational injury or airway compromise: stridor, shortness of breath, hoarse voice, soot in nose, singed nose hairs, carbonaceous sputum. Examine site, depth and distribution of burn. Check whole of body surface area. Look for circumferential burns.

Partial thickness: Subdivided into superficial and deep. Red and oedematous skin in a superficial burn, blistering and mottling in deep dermal burns; both are painful.

Full thickness: Destruction of both epidermis and dermis. Charred leathery eschar, firm and painless with loss of sensation.

Size of burn (% body surface area): Use Wallace's 'Rule of Nines' (arm or head 9%, anterior or posterior trunk 18%, leg 18%, palm area 1% and perineum 1%) or Lund–Browder chart (for children).

PATHOLOGY/PATHOGENESIS
Superficial partial thickness burns involve damage to the epidermis, healing occurs within 7 days with subsequent peeling of dead skin. Deep partial burns extend into dermis, but sweat and sebaceous glands are spared and healing occurs by epithelial regrowth over 3 weeks, usually without scarring unless infection develops. Full thickness burns involve complete destruction of all skin layers and require skin grafting, or healing will occur by scarring and contractures.

INVESTIGATIONS
Bloods: O_2 saturations, arterial blood gases and carboxyhaemoglobin if an inhalational injury. FBC, U&Es and G&S or crossmatch in severe burns.

In electrical burns: Creatine kinase, urine myoglobin for muscle damage and ECG.

MANAGEMENT
Emergency: ABCs: Secure airway, give oxygen, early endotracheal intubation may be necessary if inhalational injury. Assess of size of burn, if >15% body surface area (10% in children), IV fluids are required to prevent hypovolaemic shock. Fluid requirements can be estimated using the following:
- the Muir and Barclay formula [(% burn × weight, kg)/2] = fluid (ml) per time period (each 4 hours from time of burn for 12 hours, then each 6 hours for 12 hours and then over 12 hours); or
- the Parkland formula [4 ml × weight (kg) × % burn, with half the volume given over first 8 hours, the other half over next 16 hours].

Burn should be covered with a sterile dressing, tetanus prophylaxis and analgesia given. Antibiotics are not given prophylactically (risk of resistance developing). Nutritional support in severe burns due to intensely catabolic state. Early physiotherapy to prevent development of contractures. Consider transfer to specialist unit.

Surgery: *Escharotomy*: This is the longitudinal incision over circumferential burns to release constrictions that may compromise chest movement or limb perfusion.

Skin grafting: For full thickness or deep partial thickness once stable.

COMPLICATIONS

Early: Respiratory distress, hypothermia, myocardial depression, rhabdomyolysis, infection, e.g. *Streptococcus, Pseudomonas,* compartment syndrome, peptic ulcers (Curling's ulcer) or erosive gastritis.

Late: Hypertrophic scars and contractures.

PROGNOSIS

Depends on the depth and extent of the burn, age and the development of complications (mortality risk approximately equal to sum of age and % burn).

Gangrene and necrotising fasciitis

DEFINITION

Gangrene is tissue necrosis, either wet with superimposed infection, dry (with desiccation) or gas gangrene.

Necrotising fasciitis is a life-threatening infection that spreads rapidly along fascial planes. Fournier's gangrene is necrotising fasciitis of the perineum.

AETIOLOGY

Gangrene: Tissue ischaemia and infarction, physical trauma, thermal injury, inadvertent arterial injection, e.g. thiopentone and infection. Gas gangrene is caused by *Clostridia perfringens*.

Necrotising fasciitis: Infection with Group A streptococcus or polymicrobial with streptococci, staphylococci, bacteroides and coliforms or clostridial forms. Please see **Associations/Risk Factors** and **Pathology/Pathogenesis**.

ASSOCIATIONS/RISK FACTORS

Diabetes, peripheral vascular disease and leg ulcers, malignancy, immunosupression and steroid use are risk factors. Necrotising fasciitis occasionally occurs without obvious predisposing factor or in relation to puncture wounds, ulcers or surgical wounds.

EPIDEMIOLOGY

Gangrene is relatively common but gas gangrene and necrotising fasciitis are uncommon.

HISTORY

Gangrene: Pain with discolouration in the affected area, often the extremities or areas subject to pressure.

Necrotising fasciitis: Pain, often severe and out of proportion to the apparent physical signs. History of risk factors or predisposing event (e.g. trauma, ulcer and surgery).

EXAMINATION

Gangrene: The painful area is usually the erythematous region around the gangrenous tissue, with the latter black because of haemoglobin breakdown products, dead and insensate. The junction between the live and the dead tissues is known as the line of demarcation. In wet gangrene, the tissue becomes boggy and there may be associated pus, with a strong odour caused by anaerobes. In gas gangrene, spreading infection and destruction of tissues and muscle cause overlying oedema, discolouration and crepitus due to gas formation.

Necrotising fasciitis: Area of erythema and oedema, areas of haemorrhagic blisters may be present with crepitus on palpation. Associated signs of systemic inflammatory response and sepsis: pyrexia, tachycardia, tachypnoea and hypotension.

PATHOLOGY/PATHOGENESIS

■ *Gangrene*: Tissue damage and ischaemia predispose to colonisation and proliferation of bacteria. In the presence of an anaerobic environment, synergy between organisms occurs perpetuating the cycle of tissue damage and bacterial growth. *C. perfringens*, *C. novyi* and *C. septicum* are gram-positive rod-shaped spore-forming saprophytes. They grow in the anaerobic environment of damaged tissue and produce exotoxins, e.g. α-lethicinase, which destroys the local microcirculation, cause necrosis, haemolysis and sepsis.

■ *Necrotising fasciitis*: Most commonly a synergistic polymicrobial infection spreading along fascial planes. Often caused by Group A β-haemolytic *Streptococcus pyogenes*, or gram-negative and anaerobic synergistic infection, e.g. enterococci and bacteroides.

INVESTIGATIONS

Bloods: FBC, U&Es, glucose, CRP and blood culture.

Wound swab, pus/fluid aspirate: Microscopy, Gram stain, culture and sensitivity.

Radiography or CT-scan: May show gas in the tissues formed by organisms.

MANAGEMENT

Gangrene: Fluid resuscitation, broad-spectrum IV antibiotics with prompt surgical debridement of all pus and necrotic tissues.

Necrotising fasciitis: Aggressive debridement of all infected tissues is necessary to limit spread and systemic sepsis together with broad-spectrum antibiotics (e.g. penicillin, aminoglycoside and metronidazole). Frequent review of the wound is necessary as the need for repeated debridement is not uncommon.

Amputation: Indicated if the limb is not salvageable or gangrene is rapidly progressive.

COMPLICATIONS

Tissue destruction, limb loss, systemic inflammatory response syndrome, sepsis, septic shock and multiple organ dysfunction syndrome, death.

PROGNOSIS

Variable. If gangrenous limb is amputated early, recovery is good. Diabetes and poor peripheral vasculature are poor prognostic indicators. Gas gangrene and necrotising fasciitis are associated with high morbidity and mortality.

Lymphoedema

DEFINITION

Excessive accumulation of lymphatic fluid in the extracellular space due to impaired function of the lymphatic system.

AETIOLOGY

Primary (hereditary): In most families, the gene mutations are unknown.
Those identified include:

- *Milroy's disease*: Autosomal dominant inheritance with mutation in the vascular endothelial growth factor receptor *VEGFR-3* gene.
- *Lymphoedema distichiasis syndrome*: Inactivating mutation in transcription factor FOXC2 gene. Associated with supplementary rows of eyelashes.
- *Hypotrichosis-lymphoedema-telangiectasia syndrome*: Mutations in the transcription factor SOX18 gene.

Secondary (acquired):

- Following obstruction or destruction of lymphatic channels, e.g. infection with *Wuchereria bancrofti* (filariasis), TB, silica.
- Post-radiotherapy or surgical excision of regional lymphatics in treatment of cancer, most commonly breast.
- Malignant infiltration of regional lymph nodes.

EPIDEMIOLOGY

Primary: Uncommon, annual incidence $\sim$1/6000–10,000; 2–3$\times$ more common in females.
Secondary: Much more common. Worldwide, the most common cause is filariasis.

HISTORY

Can present at birth (Milroy's), during puberty (lymphoedema distichiasis) or any age. Most often gradual swelling of one or both lower limbs, worse towards end of the day. In other cases, swelling is of arm or genitalia. In megalymphatics, presentation can be with leaking skin vesicles, chylothorax or chylous ascites.

EXAMINATION

Early stages, skin oedema is pitting in nature. Later, the skin becomes fibrotic, brawny and non-pitting; there may be weeping from vesicles. Ankles lose contour and toes become squared off. Thickened skin areas (condylomas) can develop.

PATHOLOGY/PATHOGENESIS

Primary/congenital lymphoedema results from hypoplasia, hyperplasia and/or insufficient function of lymphatic valves. The resulting accumulation of protein-rich fluid and oedema, often with inflammation, results in fibrosis and overgrowth of adipose and connective tissue with the ensuing extremity swelling.

INVESTIGATIONS

Isotope lymphography: [99] mTc-labelled colloid is injected subcutaneously into the first web space of the foot and the movement is measured using a gamma counter.
Contrast lymphangiography: Now rarely performed.
CT or MRI scan: Can show the changes associated with lymphoedema, e.g. cutaneous thickening or oedema in fascial planes. May show the cause if an obstructive lesion is present.
Others: Bioelectric impedance analysis or tissue/lymph node biopsy.

MANAGEMENT

Conservative: Skin or foot care, limb elevation, exercise, graduated compression stockings, complex decongestive physiotherapy (CDPT) and massage with manual lymphatic drainage or pneumatic devices. BP measurement or venesection should not be carried out from affected limbs.
Medical: Treatment of infection (e.g. antibiotics for cellulitis, antifungals for tinea pedis). Diuretics have no beneficial effects.

Surgical: Rarely used. Procedures used include liposuction with aggressive postoperative compression, Homan's operation involves creating skin flaps, excising subcutaneous tissue followed by resuturing of skin. Charles' reduction involves removal of skin and subcutaneous tissue, followed by skin grafting.

COMPLICATIONS
↑ Fluid and protein renders skin prone to cellulitis, poor cosmesis, pain due to tissue swelling, reduced mobility, ulceration.

PROGNOSIS
Primary lymphoedema: Good, usually responds to conservative measures.
Secondary lymphoedema: Depends on the aetiology.

Melanoma, malignant

DEFINITION

Malignancy arising from neoplastic transformation of melanocytes, the pigment forming cells of the skin. The leading cause of death from skin disease. Can also arise in the eye, ear, GI tract or leptomeninges.

AETIOLOGY

Multifactorial, with accumulation of genetic mutations resulting in neoplastic transformation. Family history (10%), inherited mutations identified in CDKN2A and CDK4 (tumour suppressor genes) in rare familial melanoma syndrome (autosomal dominant). Congenital, e.g. xeroderma pigmentosum.

Four histopathological types:

(1) *Superficial spreading (70%)*: Typically arises in a pre-existing naevus, flat or elevated brown lesion, possibly with variegate pigmentation, expands in radial fashion before vertical growth phase.

(2) *Nodular (15%)*: Arises *de novo*, aggressive, easily bleeds or ulcerates, no radial growth phase.

(3) *Lentigo maligna (10%)*: More common in elderly with sun damage, large flat lesions, follows a more indolent growth course. Usually on the face, neck or arms.

(4) *Acral lentiginous (5%)*: Arise on palms, soles and subungual areas. Most common type in non-white populations and diagnosis often delayed.

Associated with UV light exposure (sun exposure, especially history of blistering burning, use of tanning lamps, PUVA). Fair skin, increased number of dysplastic moles.

EPIDEMIOLOGY

Steadily increasing incidence, ~6000 per year diagnosed in the UK, lifetime risk 1/60 in the USA. White races have a 20× risk to non-white races. Accounts for ~4% of skin cancers, but 3/4 of skin cancer deaths.

HISTORY

Change in size, shape or colour of a pigmented skin lesion, redness, bleeding, crusting and ulceration. However, >60% do not arise from pre-existing moles.

EXAMINATION

ABCDE criteria for examining moles:

A   Asymmetry
B   Border irregularity/bleeding
C   Colour variation
D   Diameter >6 mm
E   Elevation/evolving changes over time

Amelanotic melanoma is non-pigmented, often associated with nodular subtype or metastases of undifferentiated melanoma to the skin.

INVESTIGATIONS

Excisional biopsy: For histological diagnosis and determination of Clark's levels or Breslow thickness.

Sentinel lymph node biopsy: Sentinel lymph nodes are identified by lymphoscintigraphy and blue dye, and histologically examined for metastatic involvement.

Staging: Imaging by CT or MRI, CXR and PET scanning.

Bloods: LFTs and LDH (liver is a common site of metastases).

MANAGEMENT

Primary prevention: Limit sun overexposure, avoid sunburn, public education.

Surgical: Wide local excision, margin dependent on depth of invasion (<1 mm: 1 cm, 1–4 mm: 2 cm margin). Skin grafting may be required. Sentinel lymph node biopsy is performed if melanoma >1 mm, and if positive, a completion lymph node dissection is performed. Following treatment, careful follow-up is warranted.

Metastatic disease: Chemotherapy: relatively resistant. Response in trials to dacarbazine in combination with cisplatin and paclitaxel. Should be part of a trial. Trials have shown immunotherapy with high-dose interferon α-2b improves relapse-free but not overall survival (for high-risk tumours >4 mm and regional lymph node metastases). Studies on melanoma vaccines are under progress.

COMPLICATIONS

Local: Bleeding, ulceration.

Metastases: Bleeding, mass effect.

Post-surgical: Wound problems or lymphoedema may result after block dissection of lymph nodes.

PROGNOSIS

Five-year survival, 90–95% for lesions <1 mm depth, 13–69% with node-positive disease and median survival of 9 months with metastatic disease. Ulceration reduces survival at each tumour stage.

Poorer prognostic indicators: Ulceration, ↑ mitotic rate, trunk lesions compared to limb. Males have poorer prognosis than females.

Pressure sores

DEFINITION

An area of damage to skin and underlying tissue caused by pressure, shear and/or friction, typically over bony prominences.

AETIOLOGY

When external pressure exceeds capillary filling pressure (32 mmHg), tissue perfusion is impaired resulting in ischaemia, acidosis and waste product accumulation. Early signs of tissue damage occur in the dermis with non-blanching erythema indicating perivascular haemorrhage from capillaries. With time, there is cell death and tissue necrosis in the dermis, subcutaneous tissue and then epidermis.

ASSOCIATIONS/RISK FACTORS

- *Extrinsic*: Pressure, shear, friction and moisture.
- *Intrinsic*: Age, immobility, sensory impairment, incontinence, protein-calorie malnutrition (for each 10 g/L ↓ in albumin, threefold ↑ in risk), comorbidity and previous pressure damage.

EPIDEMIOLOGY

Common, 3–10% of hospitalised patients and nursing home residents, with >70% in those aged >70 years, with annual costs (mostly nursing time) estimated over £2.1 billion in the UK.

HISTORY

Area of erythema or ulcer may be noticed by carer, less frequently the patient may complain of pain in the affected area. Predisposing factors. The injury responsible may have occurred early on in a hospital stay, e.g. while on operating table, with the majority developing within the first 2 weeks.

EXAMINATION

Vulnerable areas are over the sacrum, coccyx, ischial tuberosities, greater trochanter, malleoli and heels, also the occiput and scapulae.

- *Stage I*: Non-blanching erythema with intact epidermis.
- *Stage II*: Shallow ulcer involving dermis (can be a blister).
- *Stage III*: Full thickness of dermis, extending into subcutaneous tissue.
- *Stage IV*: Extending beyond deep fascia into tendon, bone, muscle or joint.

This system cannot be used to measure progression or healing (e.g. Stage IV ulcers do not always start and progress through Stages I, II and III).

Colonisation of wounds by bacteria is common and unavoidable; however, infection should only be diagnosed if there is associated erythema, odour, purulent exudates or systemic signs (e.g. fever).

INVESTIGATIONS

Wound swab, blood cultures if infection suspected.

Plain radiographs, bone or [67]Gallium scans, MRI or needle bone biopsy if underlying osteomyelitis is suspected.

MANAGEMENT

Prevention is the key: Risk assessment (e.g. Waterlow scores), assessing nutritional status, avoiding excessive bed rest.

Pressure reduction: Turning the patient every 2 hours. Avoiding pressure on vulnerable sites, especially sacrum, trochanters and heels, pressure-reducing devices (static or dynamic) such as foam or air mattresses that distribute the pressure between the patient and the bed.

Wound management: Pressure reduction. Assessing severity, debridement of necrotic tissue and optimising wound environment to promote granulation and re-epithelialisation. Use of appropriate dressings that provide moisture balance, bacterial balance and debridement (e.g. hydrocolloid, hydrogel or alginates). Prevention and treatment of infection, attention to nutrition (Vitamin C and zinc supplementation in those who are deficient).

Surgical: Restricted to Stage III or IV ulcers. Debridement of necrotic material and reconstruction of affected area with myocutaneous flaps (have a high complication rate, hence attention to pre-op optimisation and post-op care are vital).

COMPLICATIONS

Infection (e.g. cellulitis or osteomyelitis), chronic ulceration, tendency to recur.

PROGNOSIS

Pressure ulcers are difficult to heal, Stage III may take several weeks of care, while only 1/3 of Stage IV have healed after 6 months; hence, prevention is key.

Squamous cell carcinoma (skin)

DEFINITION
Malignancy of the epidermal keratinocytes of the skin. Marjolin's ulcer is a squamous cell carcinoma that arises in an area of chronically inflamed/scarred skin.

AETIOLOGY
The main aetiological risk factor is UV radiation from sunlight exposure, actinic keratoses (sun-induced precancerous lesions). Others include radiation, carcinogens (like tar derivatives, cigarette smoke, soot, industrial oils and arsenic), chronic skin disease (e.g. lupus and leukoplakia), human papilloma virus, long-term immunosuppression (e.g. transplant recipients and HIV patients) and DNA repair genetic defects (xeroderma pigmentosum).

EPIDEMIOLOGY
Second most common cutaneous malignancy (20% of skin cancers). Often occurring in middle-aged and elderly light-skinned individuals. Annual incidence is about 1/4000. Male > female (2–3 : 1).

HISTORY
Skin lesion, ulcerated, recurrent bleeding or non-healing.

EXAMINATION
Variable appearance: Ulcerated, hyperkeratotic, crusted or scaly, non-healing, lesion, often on sun-exposed areas. Palpate for local lymphadenopathy.

PATHOLOGY/PATHOGENESIS
Bowen's disease is intraepidermal carcinoma *in situ* (intraepidermal proliferation of atypical keratinocytes, basement membrane is intact), visable as solitary or multiple red-brown scaly patches. In squamous cell carcinoma, the malignant keratinocytes invade locally into the dermis and can spread to local lymph nodes and distally metastasise, e.g. lungs and liver. Staging is based on the TNM system.

INVESTIGATIONS
Skin biopsy: Confirms malignancy and distinguishes it from other skin lesions.
Fine-needle aspiration or lymph node biopsy: Only necessary if suspicion of metastasis.
Staging: CT and/or MRI, PET scanning.

MANAGEMENT
Surgical: For Bowen's disease, curettage and cryotherapy, cauterisation or photodynamic therapy can be sufficient to eradicate lesion. Invasive squamous cell carcinomas should be excised with an appropriate margin of 4 or 6 mm (low- or high-risk lesions).
Mohs' micrographic surgery: Excision with close margins and histological examination during surgery to confirm complete excision. Can be used in areas where large excisions are difficult, e.g. lips and near eyes.
Sentinal lymph node biopsy: Can be performed where there is risk of metastatic spread.
Local radiotherapy: For larger lesions or if surgery is difficult (cure rate lower compared to surgery).
Medical: Topical 5-fluorouracil for Bowen's disease or intralesional interferons if other options are difficult. Chemotherapy is used for metastatic disease.

COMPLICATIONS
Sun-exposed skin squamous cell carcinomas are usually local at the time of diagnosis, but 1/3 of those on lips or lingual membranes have spread by the time of diagnosis.

PROGNOSIS
Good if treated appropriately. High-risk factors include: (1) tumour location (lips, ears and scar); (2) tumour size >2 cm (1.5 cm on lips and ear); (3) deep level of invasion; (4) poorly differentiated; (5) perineural invasion and (6) recurrent tumours.

Abdominal aortic aneurysm repair (open)

INDICATIONS
Elective: Large asymptomatic aneurysms (>5.5 cm in diameter).
Expanding aneurysms (>0.5 cm in 1 year).
Emergency: Leaking or ruptured aneurysms. Symptomatic aneurysms.

ANATOMY
An abdominal aortic aneurysm is an abnormal focal dilatation of the abdominal aorta. Ninety-five percent arise below the renal artery origin and can extend to include the iliac arteries. Typically fusiform in shape, they expand (rate of 0.2–0.8 cm/year) with the risk of rupture depending on diameter. Laminated thrombus accumulates within the aneurysm that has the potential to embolise distally.

INVESTIGATIONS
In elective repairs: Aneurysm size and anatomy is assessed by ultrasound and CT/MRA scanning. 3D CT reconstruction allows endovascular planning.
Pre-op: FBC, clotting, U&Es, crossmatch (six to eight units of blood), CXR, ECG, Echo or cardio-pulmonary testing.
Post-op: Close monitoring HDU/ITU setting. Inspect lower limbs for emboli. DVT prophylaxis.

PROCEDURE
Access: Either a full length midline laparotomy or a transverse incision which allows better epidural pain control. Rarely performed as hand-assisted laparoscopic repair.
Exposure: The small bowel is displaced upwards to the right, exposing the retroperitoneum over the aorta, which is incised slightly to the right to prevent damage to the left sympathetic chain. Dissection is carried out to expose the aorta from the infrarenal aorta to the bifurcation, with care taken to avoid injury to the left renal vein, which crosses in front of the aorta. The inferior mesenteric artery is identified, ligated and divided. Systemic heparin is administered and clamps are placed at the proximal and distal ends of the aneurysm.
Opening the aneurysm: The aneurysm is opened longitudinally, exposing the contents. Thrombus within the aneurysm is removed, and any bleeding from lumbar arteries in the back wall is controlled with sutures.
Insertion of graft: The walls of the distal aorta and bifurcation are inspected. In an aneurysm confined to the aorta, a tube graft is used. If the distal aorta or proximal iliacs are diseased, an aorto-iliac, or more rarely, aorto-bifemoral trouser graft is used. The grafts are sutured in place with prolene sutures and flushed to remove air or debris.
Assessment of graft: The aortic clamp is gradually released ensuring haemostasis, followed by gradual opening of the distal end with close monitoring due to the risk of hypotension and arrythmias. The aneurysm sac is then closed around the graft and sutured to prevent adhesions with the anastomosis suture line.
Closure: Mass closure with clips or sutures to skin.
In emergency setting of aneurysm rupture, the patient is rushed to theatre, maintaining systolic BP of ~80–100 mmHg. The patient is rapidly prepared and draped with surgery commencing immediately following a 'crash induction' of anaesthesia. The aim is for rapid clamping and control of the bleeding vessel.

COMPLICATIONS
Haemorrhage, myocardial ischaemia, MI or arrhythmias, CVA, respiratory complications (atelectasis, infection and ARDS), colonic ischaemia, spinal ischaemia, atheromatous

Abdominal aortic aneurysm repair (open) (continued)

embolisation, renal failure, graft thrombosis, endoleak. *Late:* Graft infection, aorto-enteric fistula, false aneurysm at anastomosis.

PROGNOSIS

Elective operative mortality is now <5% in most units. Emergency repair of a leaking or ruptured aortic aneurysm has a very high mortality.

Amputation, above knee

INDICATIONS

Ischaemia, infarction or gangrene: Acute or chronic lower limb ischaemia or caused by severe trauma or burns.

Malignancy: Certain tumours (e.g. osteosarcoma).

Severe infection: Gas gangrene (*Clostridium perfringens*) or necrotising fasciitis.

Rare: Intractable ulceration or painful paralysed limbs.

ANATOMY

AKA: At the level of 15 cm above the tibial plateau is optimal.

Through-knee amputation: Sometimes indicated (e.g. if there has been prior orthopaedic fixation of femur), disadvantage is unpredictable healing of skin flaps and a bulbous stump for prosthesis fitting.

Gritti–Stokes amputation: Involves femur division at the supracondylar level, leaving a longer stump than AKA and ↑ stability for the patient while sitting.

Others (e.g. disarticulation of hip and hindquarter amputation): These are rarely performed, and mainly for severe infection or malignancy.

INVESTIGATIONS

Pre-op: Ideally, multidisciplinary assessment including surgical, anaesthetic and prosthetic specialists. Assessment of the level of amputation, given severity of disease and patient factors (e.g. rehabilitation prospects). Insulin sliding scale if diabetic, appropriate blood tests and crossmatch blood, urinary catheterisation if appropriate.

Post-op: Rehabilitation with early physiotherapy, early walking aids (e.g. pneumatic post-amputation mobility aid) or prosthesis fitting.

PROCEDURE

Access: Two equal fish mouth-shaped skin flaps are marked on the skin, with their upper ends at the level of femur transaction. This is ~15 cm above the tibial plateau.

Muscle and vessel ligation: During skin incision, the long saphenous vein is ligated and the muscles of the anterior and posterior thigh compartments are divided by diathermy. Vastus lateralis is sutured to the adductors, and quadriceps to the hamstrings. Arteries and veins are ligated and nerves are divided cleanly under gentle traction.

Bone amputation: The femur is stripped of periosteum and divided, with filing of bone ends to create a smooth surface.

Closure: Once haemostasis is achieved, the two myoplastic flaps are brought together and the skin is closed with sutures. A drain may be left *in situ*.

COMPLICATIONS

Early: Pain, DVT, flap ischaemia, stump haematoma, neuroma or infection, stump length too long or short, bony spurs, psychological problems; ~15% early mortality.

Late: 'Phantom' limb pain (reduced by strong analgesia post-op), neuroma formation, erosion of bone through skin, ischaemia, osteomyelitis, ulceration.

PROGNOSIS

Amputations are most often carried out in those with concomitant severe atherosclerotic disease and there is a major risk of other vascular problems with survival only 30% at 5 years post-amputation.

For diagrammatic review on general amputations, see Fig. 20.

Amputation, below knee

INDICATIONS

Ischaemia, infarction or gangrene: Acute or chronic lower limb ischaemia, severe trauma or burns.

Malignancy: Certain tumours (e.g. osteosarcoma and malignant melanoma).

Severe infection: Gas gangrene (*Clostridium perfringens*) or necrotising fasciitis.

Rare: Intractable ulceration or painful paralysed limbs.

ANATOMY

Below knee: Two techniques for transtibial amputation: Burgess long posterior flap and Robinson's skew flap techniques.

Ankle level: Seldom performed due to difficulty attaching prosthesis.

Midfoot: Lisfranc's involving disarticulation between tarsal and metatarsal bones or Chopart's disarticulation of the talonavicular and calcaneocuboid joints.

Ray: Involves excision of a toe by division through the metatarsal bone.

Toe: Division is through the proximal phalanx, as cutting through a joint exposes avascular cartilage that does not heal well.

INVESTIGATIONS

Pre-op: Ideally, multidisciplinary assessment including surgical, anaesthetic, prosthetic specialists, physiotherapists, psychologists, etc. Assessment of the level of amputation given severity of disease and patient factors (e.g. rehabilitation prospects). Insulin sliding scale if diabetic, appropriate blood tests and crossmatch blood, urinary catheterisation if appropriate.

Post-op: Rehabilitation with early physiotherapy, early walking aids (e.g. pneumatic post-amputation mobility aid) or prosthesis fitting.

PROCEDURE

Access: Skin flaps are marked on the skin prior to incision with a longer posterior flap (Burgess) or skew anteromedial and posterolateral flaps. The level of tibial transaction is ~14 cm below knee joint or 10–12 cm below tibial tuberosity.

Ligation of muscle and vessels: During skin incision, the long saphenous vein is ligated and the muscles of the anterior and peroneal compartments are divided by diathermy. Arteries and veins are ligated and, following diathermy of accompanying vasa nervorum, the tibial nerve is divided cleanly under gentle traction.

Bone amputation: The fibula is divided 2 cm proximally following stripping of periosteum. The tibia is also stripped and divided, with filing of bone ends to a smooth surface.

Closure: The posterior flap includes some gastrocnemius muscle to cover the cut tibia, forming a cylindrical stump. After haemostasis is achieved, the skin is closed with sutures. A drain may be left *in situ*.

COMPLICATIONS

Early: Pain, DVT, flap ischaemia, stump haematoma, neuroma or infection, stump length too long or short, bony spurs, psychological problems.

Late: 'Phantom' limb pain (reduced by good analgesia post-op), neuroma formation, erosion of bone through skin, ischaemia, osteomyelitis, ulceration.

PROGNOSIS

Amputations are most often carried out in those with concomitant severe atherosclerotic disease and there is major risk of other vascular problems with survival only 30% at 5 years.

For diagrammatic review on general amputations, see Fig. 20.

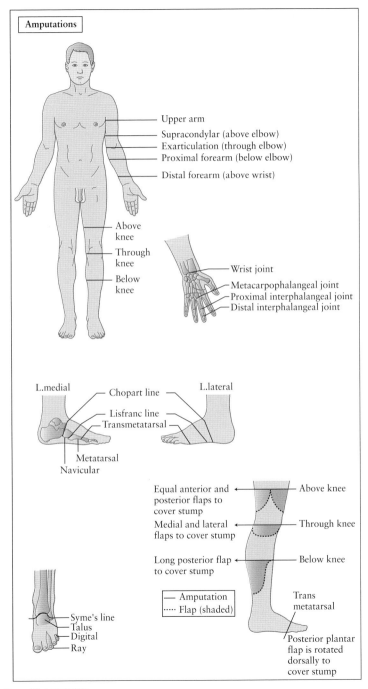

Figure 20 Amputations.

Appendicectomy

INDICATIONS

Acute appendicitis. Interval procedure following management of an appendix mass with IV antibiotics.

ANATOMY

The appendix arises at the convergence of the taeniae coli on the posteromedial side of the caecum, 2.5 cm below the junction with the terminal ileum. The length varies from 1.2 to 22.0 cm and the appendix can lie in variable positions, retrocaecal ($\sim$70%), pelvic (20%), subcaecal (2%) and pre- or post-ileal (5%). It has a mesentery, the mesoappendix, in which runs the appendicular artery, a branch of the ileocolic artery. Lymphatics from the appendix traverse the mesoappendix to drain into ileocaecal nodes.

INVESTIGATIONS

Pre-op: FBC, U&Es, LFT, amylase, CRP and urinalysis (for investigation of abdominal pain). In females of childbearing age, a pregnancy test should be performed. Antibiotic are started if there are signs of sepsis, otherwise a single prophylactic dose is given at the time of surgery.

Post-op: Antibiotics may be continued if the appendix is inflamed. DVT prophlyaxis.

PROCEDURE

Can be performed laparoscopically or open.

Always examine the patient on the table to see if a mass is present.

Access: Lanz (horizontal skin crease) incision, centred on McBurney's point (2/3 the distance from umbilicus to anterior superior iliac spine), the subcutaneous fat is divided and external oblique aponeurosis exposed. A small slit is made in the direction of the fibres, then extended with scissors. Internal oblique muscle is split along the direction of its fibres by blunt dissection, as is transversus, and the opening is gently enlarged using retractors. Once the peritoneum is exposed, it is gently picked up with a clip. A second clip is then placed and the first clip repositioned. Palpate to ensure there is no bowel caught between the clips before a small cut is made, and then extended.

Identification: The peritoneal cavity is inspected for free fluid or pus. The caecum is identified and the taeniae are followed to find the base of the appendix, freeing it from inflammatory adhesions by gentle blunt dissection. Babcock's forceps is used to pick up the appendix. If the appendix is found to be normal ('lily-white'), it should still be removed, however, the small bowel should be systematically inspected for terminal ileitis, a Meckel's diverticulum or mesenteric adenitis. In females, the right ovary and tube should be inspected.

Resection: The mesoappendix is clipped and divided after tying off, ensuring haemostasis. A crushing clamp is used to crush the base of the appendix and the base is transfixed or tied before removal. The appendix is sent for histological analysis. Usually the appendix stump is buried using a purse string suture. The cavity should be washed if there has been inflammatory fluid or pus.

Closure: The incision is then closed in layers. A continuous suture of the peritoneum, interrupted sutures to the muscle layers and then continuous sutures to the external oblique (the latter is very important in preventing subsequent hernias) are performed. A subcuticular absorbable suture is usually used for the skin. Local anaesthetic infiltration reduces post-op pain.

Laparoscopic appendicectomy: An alternative technique, which is very useful in women where the diagnosis may be equivocal as it can be both diagnostic and therapeutic. Following capnoperitoneum and port placement, the mesoappendix is divided from the appendix and loop suturing or endostapling across the appendix base before excision and removal through a port.

COMPLICATIONS

Relatively uncommon, but presence reflects the degree of inflammation or peritonitis, e.g. ileus, haemorrhage, wound infection, more rarely, local abscess or a pelvic abscess.

PROGNOSIS

Usually good with mortality <1% but this can be higher in elderly or if perforation occurs.

Bariatric surgery

INDICATIONS

Severe obesity, where lifestyle measures ± medical therapy has not been effective. NICE or NIH guidelines are:

- BMI $\geq$40 kg/m^2; or
- BMI 35–40 kg/m^2 with obesity-related comorbidities (e.g. hypertension, Type II diabetes, hyperlipidaemia and obstructive sleep apnoea).

Patients must undergo multidisciplinary assessment, be fit for anaesthesia, understand consequences of surgery and commit to long-term follow-up.

Contraindications: Inflammatory bowel disease, chronic pancreatitis, cirrhosis, drug or alcohol abuse or psychiatric illness.

ANATOMY

Divided into restrictive (limit intake), malabsorptive or combination procedures, but mechanisms may be more complex, e.g. reduced ghrelin production by the gastric fundus in sleeve gastrectomy (see Fig. 21a–21c).

Gastric restriction: Laparoscopic adjustable gastric band, sleeve gastrectomy.

Restriction with some intestinal malabsorption: Roux-en-Y gastric bypass.

Malabsorptive with some restriction: Biliopancreatic diversion with/without duodenal switch.

INVESTIGATIONS

Pre-procedure: Multidisciplinary workup, cardiopulmonary, endocrine and psychiatric assessment and dietician input. Liquid diet 2 weeks prior to surgery to reduce the size of liver and facilitate surgery *Bloods:* FBC, U&E, LFTs, lipids, TFT, iron, B12, folate and crossmatching of blood.

Post-procedure: Gastric bypass, biliopancreatic diversion: Oral contrast study to assess for leak (optional), dietician review and initial liquid diet, building up slowly, lifelong vitamin and mineral supplementation, monitoring and follow-up.

PROCEDURE

Open or laparoscopic.

Gastric band: Adjustable silicone band is placed around the upper stomach creating a 15–20 ml pouch. Band tightness can be adjusted by saline inflation through a port in subcutaneous tissue.

Roux-en-Y gastric bypass: Stomach is divided, creating a 15–30 ml pouch that is connected to the jejunum via a Roux-en-Y gastrojejunostomy.

Biliopancreatic diversion: Partial gastrectomy, with the gastric remnant anastomosed to the distal ileum 50–100 cm from the ileocaecal valve, the segment where absorption occurs. In the duodenal switch procedure, the first part of the duodenum and pylorus are left intact, decreasing the incidence of dumping syndrome and stomal ulceration.

Benefits: Weight loss (gastric band: ~50% excess weight can be lost, 70% for malabsorptive procedures). Reduction in comorbidities such as diabetes, hypertension, reduction in overall mortality, reduction in some malignancies, improved mobility and self-esteem. Following weight loss, many require body contouring surgery to remove redundant skin.

COMPLICATIONS

Short-term: *General*: Bleeding, infection, anastomotic leaks, DVT/PE, arrhythmias, 30-day mortality <1%. *Specific:* Gastric band slippage, migration, erosion. *Gastric Roux-en-Y bypass:* Dumping syndrome, ulcers, internal herniation, nausea and vomiting due to over-eating.

Long-term: Anastomotic stenosis, marginal ulceration, internal herniation, gallstones, malabsorption, nutritional deficiencies, e.g. iron, calcium, fat soluble vitamins, thiamine, B12, copper, neurological symptoms, bone demineralisation, protein-calorie malnutrition, failure (of weight loss or weight regain, 5–10%).

(a)

(b)

(c)

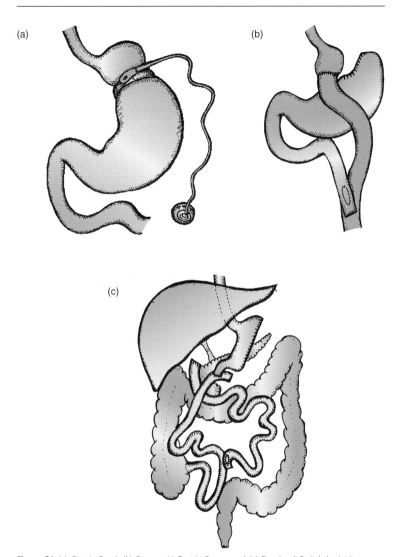

Figure 21 (a) Gastric Band, (b) Roux-en-Y Gastric Bypass and (c) Duodenal Switch bariatric surgery procedures.

Cardiac transplantation

INDICATIONS

Idiopathic cardiomyopathy and ischaemic heart disease (~99%).

Congenital heart disease, valvular cardiac disease and myocarditis (~1%).

Recipient criteria:

- End-stage heart disease with a life expectancy of <1 year.
- Absence of hepatic or renal failure.
- Absence of active systemic infection or malignancy.
- Psychosocial stability, able to comply with immunosuppressive therapy and follow-up care.

ANATOMY

Orthotopic transplantation: The donor heart replaces most of the recipient's heart. The latter is removed, excising the ventricles, but leaving the great vessels, right and left atrium. The donor heart is anastomosed to the left atria, then right atria and then great vessels. Alternatively, a bicaval anastamosis can be performed (reduced atrial and valvular problems).

Heterotopic transplantation: The recipient's heart is not removed and the donor heart is placed parallel to the recipient's. Less commonly performed. Donor heart assists recipient's own heart. Can be performed in pulmonary hypertension.

INVESTIGATIONS

Pre-op: Extensive multidisciplinary workup including infection screening, blood testing, blood grouping, panel-reactive antibody and tissue typing. Anaesthetic assessment. *Imaging:* Coronary angiography, echo and CXR. Pulmonary function tests. Assessment of pulmonary vascular resistance and maximal venous oxygen consumption (MVO_2, a predictor of severity of heart failure).

Donors: ABO compatible heart beating with brain stem death criteria met. Should be free from cardiac pathology. Donor surgery is performed by a specialist team. Preservation times tolerated by the heart are short (up to ~6 hours).

Post-op: Patients are initially managed in intensive care with close monitoring. Immunosuppressive therapy (e.g. cyclosporin or azathioprine) is given. Endomyocardial biopsies are used to assess for graft rejection.

PROCEDURE (OTHOTOPIC)

Access: Median sternotomy.

Cardiopulmonary bypass: It is used to oxygenate and circulate blood during surgery on the heart.

Recipient organ removal: An incision is made through both atria of the recipient's heart at mid-atrial level. The ascending aorta is divided and the pulmonary artery is divided just before the branching into the left and right pulmonary artery. The recipient's heart is removed.

Donor organ preparation: The heart is carefully prepared for implantation.

Recipient transplantation (inflow anastomosis): The left atrium is anastomosed to the remnant of the recipient's left atria with running sutures. Topical cooling with iced saline slush is applied to the donor heart externally to keep it cool. The right atrium is then anastomosed to the remnant of the recipient's right atria.

Restoring circulation (and outflow anastomosis): Systemic rewarming is started while the aorta and the pulmonary artery anastomosis are performed. Sinus rhythm returns spontaneously or is reinstituted by cardioversion. The patient is gradually taken off the bypass circuit allowing the heart to fill and resume cardiac ejection. On satisfactory cardiac output, all cannulae are removed.

Closure: Temporary pacing wires are inserted into the atrium and/or ventricles with two thoracostomy drains inserted in the pericardium and chest cavity. The sternum is closed with interrupted steel wires and the skin is closed.

COMPLICATIONS
Early: Bleeding, infection, organ dysfunction, acute rejection, renal failure, arrhythmias.
Late: Infection, valve regurgitation, accelerated coronary artery disease, chronic rejection, hypertension, post-transplantation maligancy.

PROGNOSIS
Operative mortality rate of 3–5%. Overall 90% 1-year survival and 78% 5-year survival.

Carotid endarterectomy

INDICATIONS

(Absolute) Symptomatic carotid stenosis >70–99%.

(Relative) Symptomatic stenosis >50%, if perioperative stroke/death rate is <6%, preferably within 2 weeks of the patient's last symptoms.

(Relative) Asymptomatic men <75 years with 70–99% stenosis, if the perioperative stroke/ death risk is <3%.

ANATOMY

The right common carotid arises at the bifurcation of the innominate artery behind the right sternoclavicular joint and the left arises from the arch of the aorta. The common carotid divides (level can be variable, ~C4) into the internal carotid (which has no branches in the neck) and the external carotid that supplies the exterior skull, face and the greater part of the neck. The carotids lie beside the internal jugular vein and a number of nerves are at risk during dissection including: (1) mandibular branch of the facial nerve; (2) ansa cervicalis looping across the carotids to supply infrahyoid and geniohyoid; (3) hypoglossal nerve courses medially across the anterior aspect of the external and internal carotids to supply the tongue; (4) the vagus nerve exits the jugular foramen and courses caudally in the carotid sheath, its superior and recurrent laryngeal branches are at risk.

INVESTIGATIONS

Pre-op: Carotid duplex is first-line investigation to quantify extent of stenosis. Other imaging modalities include CT and MR angiography and digital subtraction angiography. Concomitant coronary artery disease is common, so an ECG, echocardiogram, and if necessary, coronary angiogram. Pre-, peri- and postoperative aspirin and statin should be given.

Post-op: Frequent neurologic assessment should be carried out as well as haemodynamic and ECG monitoring. Observe for bleeding that may compromise the airway.

Follow-up care: Management of cardiovascular risk factors. Carotid duplex can be performed at variable intervals to monitor for restenosis or contralateral stenosis.

PROCEDURE

Anaesthesia: Can be performed under general or local anaesthesia, both are safe (GALA trial). The latter offers the advantage of allowing direct evaluation of the patient's neurological status without sophisticated monitoring. Under GA, monitoring of cerebral blood flow can be performed by EEG, stump pressures or transcranial Doppler.

Incision: An oblique incision is made along the anterior border of the sternocleidomastoid muscle. Preoperative marking or localisation of the carotid bifurcation can be helpful.

Dissection of the common, internal and external carotid arteries: Careful handling and dissection of vessels to avoid triggering embolism. Also avoiding injury to the internal jugular vein and its tributaries, hypoglossal and vagus nerves. Manipulation of the carotid body can trigger BP changes.

Arteriotomy: Following heparinisation, the arteries are clamped and a longitudinal arteriotomy is made from the common into the internal carotid. If required a shunt is placed, e.g. Javid or Pruitt-Inahara shunt.

Removal of plaque: The plaque is peeled away from the artery wall with an appropriate instrument, e.g. Watson Cheyne dissector, taking care to avoid intimal flaps and flushing with heparinised saline to remove debris and clots.

Closure: The arteriotomy is closed with prolene suture, removing the shunt if placed. The arteriotomy can be closed directly or with a prosthetic or vein patch. A drain is often placed until the following day.

COMPLICATIONS

Cardiac ischaemia, nerve injury (2–7%, mandibular branch of the facial nerve, recurrent laryngeal nerve or hypoglossal nerves), bleeding, hypertension, hypotension, perioperative stroke. The perioperative mortality rate is 0.5–1.8%.

Chest drain

INDICATION

Pneumothorax: Trauma, tension after needle decompression, ventilated patients, persistent or recurrent after simple aspiration.

Haemothorax: Trauma.

Pleural effusions: e.g. malignant, parapneumonic.

Postoperative: after, e.g. oesophagectomy, thoracotomy, cardiac surgery.

ANATOMY

Chest drain insertion should be placed in the 'safe triangle', bordered by the anterior border of latissimus dorsi, the lateral border of pectoralis major, apex below the axilla and above the upper border of sixth rib. Placement should be in the fourth or fifth rib space (the diaphragm rises to the fifth rib on expiration). Dissection and drain placement should be over the superior aspect of the rib to avoid injury to the intercosal nerve and vessel bundles that run below each rib.

INVESTIGATION

Tension pneumothorax: None necessary, proceed without delay to emergency decompression with a large bore cannula in the second intercostal space in the mid-clavicular line.

Pre-procedure: Imaging: CXR, occasionally CT depending on clinical scenario. Ultrasound-guided drain insertion (to guide safe placement) is useful in effusions or empyemas. Informed consent and explanation, oxygen, analgesia, correction of coagulopathy.

Post-procedure: Repeat CXR to assess tube position. Close monitoring of output/bubbling/swinging.

PROCEDURE

Positioning: Position the patient, e.g. lying back with arm abducted to provide access to the chest sidewall. Confirm correct side. Aseptic technique, clean the skin and drape.

Incision: Infiltrate local anaesthetic. Make an incision, usually just anterior to the midaxillary line at the fourth or fifth intercostal space. Blunt dissect through the intercostal muscles over the fifth or sixth rib to avoid the neurovascular bundle to enter the chest through the pleura with a palpable 'pop'.

Insertion: Insert a finger to confirm no adhesions and insert a chest drain (32–36F in trauma) mounted on a clamp if necessary. For pneumothorax, drain is aimed apically and for fluid basally.

Securing drain: The drain should be secured in place with a non-absorbable suture and a purse string left loosely in place to close the wound when the drain is removed. The drain is attached to an underwater seal.

Chest drain care: Clamping chest drains is almost never indicated (may lead to tension pneumthorax). Never raise the drain bottle above the patient or fluid will drain into the patient from the bottle. The meniscus in the bottle should 'swing' with each breath.

COMPLICATIONS

Damage to thoracic, mediastinal and upper abdominal structures. Haemothorax (often intercostal vessel injury – may require thoracotomy), lung laceration, diaphragmatic injury, drain placed subcutaneously, drain falling out, infection and empyema, blocked drain, recurrence after removal.

Cholecystectomy

INDICATIONS

Symptomatic gallstones.

Can be carried out in an acute setting, within 72 hours of onset of acute cholecystitis, i.e. a 'hot' gallbladder.

For open cholecystectomy: Suspected gallbladder cancer.

Conversion from laparoscopic: Inability to identify anatomy, e.g. multiple adhesions, failure to progress or intraoperative complications.

ANATOMY

The gallbladder is made up of the fundus, body, infundibulum and neck that may develop a Hartmann's pouch. The cystic duct connects the gallbladder to the junction of the common hepatic and common bile duct, and its mucosa forms folds known as the spiral valves of Heister. Anatomical variants are common. The key to dissection is Calot's triangle, made up by the lower edge of the liver, common hepatic duct medially and the cystic duct inferiorly. The cystic artery, a branch of the right hepatic artery, usually runs through here to the gallbladder. A duct of Luschka may run directly between the liver and the gallbladder.

INVESTIGATIONS

Pre-op: Ultrasound to diagnose gallstones. FBC, U&Es, LFTs and G&S are baseline blood tests.

Post-op: Laparoscopic cholecystectomy can be performed as a day case procedure. DVT prophylaxis.

PROCEDURE

Anaesthesia: General anaesthesia. Antibiotic prophylaxis if bile spillage.

Incision: Laparoscopy: The primary trocar is introduced using an open (Hassan) or closed (Veress needle) technique. A pneumoperitoneum is created by insufflation of CO_2. After inspection, three further ports, one epigastric and two along the right costal margin, are introduced under direct vision. A nasogastric tube can be used to deflate the stomach. Patient's head is tilted and right side up.

Open: A right subcostal (Kocher's) incision is performed.

Cholecystectomy: The gallbladder is grasped and retracted upwards to expose Calot's triangle. Omental and peritoneal adhesions are divided and dissection is performed to identify the cystic duct and cystic artery (vigilance is important for anatomical variation). The cystic duct is clipped near the gallbladder and an intraoperative cholangiogram can be performed to identify stones in the common bile duct if required. The cystic artery and duct are clipped proximally and distally, and divided. The gallbladder is then dissected from the undersurface of the liver. Spilled gallstones should be retrieved and removed. A subhepatic drain can be placed if concern about risk of bleeding or bile leak.

Closure: The gallbladder is placed in a bag. Following haemostasis and local lavage if necessary, the bag is extracted via a port site. The ports are removed under direct vision and the wounds are closed.

COMPLICATIONS

Early: Bleeding, bile leak, bile duct injury (increased risk if active inflammation), infection, visceral injury.

Late: Post-cholecystectomy syndrome (persistent dyspeptic symptoms), biliary stricture, port-site or incisional hernias.

Circumcision, male

INDICATIONS

Elective: Most commonly performed in infants or young boys for religious or cultural reasons. Recurrent balanoposthitis (infection of the foreskin and penis), phimosis, paraphimosis, balanitis xerotica obliterans (lichen sclerosus of the foreskin) and penile carcinoma.

Contraindications: Hypospadias, chordee and buried penis.

Emergency: Presentation with severely inflamed/infected foreskin or penis; in these cases, a dorsal slit of the phimotic foreskin is safer, as there is a risk of exacerbating infection and poor cosmesis. A formal circumcision is performed once infection and swelling have settled down.

ANATOMY

The foreskin covers and protects the glans and external urethral meatus. It consists of stratified squamous epithelium with underlying lamina propria and dartos muscle layers. Separation from the glans occurs gradually in young boys and is complete in 90% by age 5 years.

Vascular supply: Dorsal artery from the internal pudendal artery and superficial branches of the external pudendal arteries anastomose to supply the penile skin. Venous drainage is via the superficial dorsal vein that drains into the superficial external pudendal vein.

Nerve supply: Innervation is by the dorsal nerve of the penis (a branch of the pudendal nerve) and branches of the perineal nerves from S2, S3 and S4.

INVESTIGATIONS

If patient is healthy, no particular pre-op investigations are necessary.

PROCEDURE

Can be performed as a day procedure under general anaesthesia and/or caudal or local penile block.

Procedure: Most common technique involves making a dorsal slit and then dissecting and excising the foreskin with careful haemostasis. Suture of the penile skin to mucosa at the corona is carried out using interrupted absorbable sutures. A gauze dressing is placed around the wound to prevent adherence to undergarments. The foreskin is routinely sent for histological examination.

Forceps-guided circumcision (alternative method): The foreskin is pulled forward in front of the glans, a forceps is clamped across it and it is excised with a scalpel. The cut edges of the inner and outer skin are then sutured.

Plastibel circumcision: A plastic ring is placed under the foreskin introduced after dorsally slitting the foreskin. A ligature is applied over the ring and the distal tissue necroses. The ring and dead foreskin come away after a week or so.

COMPLICATIONS

Early: Haemorrhage (1–2%), penile injury (e.g. diathermy burns), urinary retention, infection.

Late: Meatal stenosis or ulcer, urethral fistula, stitch sinus, recurrent phimosis due to inadequate circumcision, chordee due to excessive skin removal.

PROGNOSIS

A commonly performed procedure usually performed for cultural reasons or benign problems.

Colorectal resections, abdomino perineal resection

INDICATIONS

Tumours of the lower rectum where the tumour is too close to the anal sphincter to achieve adequate margins or residual anal tumour post chemoradiotherapy (see Fig. 22).

ANATOMY

The rectum (12 cm) begins at the level of the third sacral vertebra, passes downward, lying in the sacrococcygeal curve, and extends anterior to the tip of the coccyx. It then bends sharply backward into the anal canal. Anteriorly is the fascia of Denonvilliers, bladder and prostate or vagina and posteriorly, the endopelvic (Waldeyer's) fascia, separating the mesorectum from the sacrum and hypogastric nerves.

Vascular: The inferior mesenteric artery supplies the upper rectum via the superior rectal artery. The middle and inferior rectal arteries supply the lower rectum and derive from the internal iliac artery. The rectal venous plexus drains into the superior, middle and inferior rectal vessels. The rectal venous plexus is a site of portacaval connection.

Lymphatics: Lymph from the upper and middle rectum drain to inferior mesenteric nodes, lower can drain to internal iliac nodes and the anus below the dentate line drains to inguinal nodes.

INVESTIGATIONS

Imaging: CT, MRI, endorectal ultrasound: For planning and assessing suitability for an abdominoperineal excision.

Colonoscopy: For tissue diagnosis and to exclude synchronous tumours.

Pre-op: Bloods, ECG, crossmatch, thromboprophylaxis, stoma marking, general anaesthetic assessment and bowel preparation.

Post-op: After elective surgery, enhanced recovery: Early return to eating and drinking, mobilisation, good analgesia, IV fluids until oral intake adequate, monitor FBC and electrolytes and urine output. Continue thromboprophylaxis, wound and stoma care, and education.

PROCEDURE

Patient is placed in the Lloyd Davies position. The anal opening is sutured shut.

Incision: Lower midline incision or can be performed laparoscopically.

Mobilisation: The left colon and sigmoid are mobilised as in a low anterior resection. The inferior mesenteric artery and vein are divided. The rectum is mobilised and dissected with total mesorectal excision to the level of the levator ani muscles. The perineal phase involves making an elliptical incision around the anus, extending posteriorly dividing the anococcygeal ligament. The incision is then deepened through muscle until connection is made with the abdominal side of the surgery. Following colon division, the anus and rectum are removed from the perineal side. An end colostomy is fashioned, usually in the left iliac fossa.

Closure: A pelvic drain can be left in situ. Mass closure of the abdominal wall, clips or sutures to skin and the perineal surface is closed with subcuticular sutures.

COMPLICATIONS

Bleeding, infection, necrosis of the stoma or perineal wound, ileus, bladder dysfunction or impotence due to nerve injury, stoma problems, hernia, DVT/PE, recurrence.

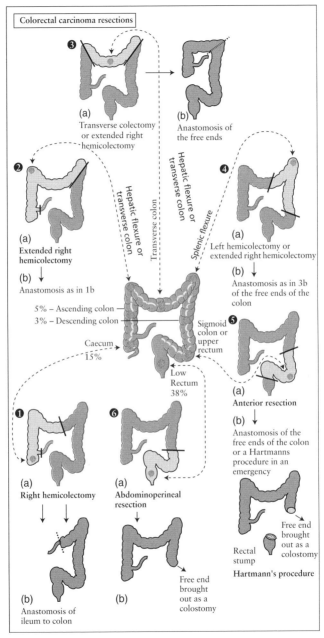

Figure 22 Colorectal carcinoma resections.

Colorectal resection, left hemicolectomy

INDICATIONS

Elective: Tumours of the descending colon and proximal sigmoid colon are the commonest indications. Severe diverticular disease.

Emergency: Occasionally indicated for obstruction, perforation, haemorrhage or ischaemia.

ANATOMY

The descending colon extends from the splenic flexure to the sigmoid colon at the pelvic brim and peritoneum covers its anterior surface and sides. The splenic flexure is attached to the diaphragm by the phrenicocolic ligament which is in continuity with the greater omentum and intimately related to the spleen and tail of the pancreas. Posteriorly is related to the left kidney, lumbar and iliac fascia.

Vascular: The inferior mesenteric artery (IMA) supplies the descending colon, the sigmoid colon and the superior 2/3 of the rectum. The left colic artery arises from the IMA and its ascending branch forms part of the marginal artery (of Drummond). Venous drainage by the inferior mesenteric vein into the portal system.

INVESTIGATIONS

Imaging: Abdominal radiograph, erect CXR, barium enema, CT scan for diagnosis and staging.

Sigmoidoscopy/colonoscopy: For diagnosis and biopsy. Endoscopic tattooing is useful to enable extraluminal localisation of colonic lesion.

Pre-op: Bloods: FBC, U&Es, clotting and crossmatch. General anaesthetic assessment. Dose of prophylactic antibiotics, thromboprophylaxis. Bowel preparation may be indicated.

Post-op: Enhanced recovery with early return to drinking and eating, mobilisation, good analgesia. Maintenance of IV fluids until oral intake adequate. An accurate record of fluid balance should be maintained. DVT prophylaxis. If signs or symptoms of post-op ileus, then revert to NG tube, IV fluids until settling. Any signs of systemic upset in the postoperative period, then an anastomotic leak needs to be excluded.

PROCEDURE

Position: Modified lithotomy/Lloyd Davis.

Access: Midline incision or laparoscopic approach. Intra-abdominal contents are assessed, e.g. for evidence of enlarged lymph nodes or liver metastases, and the small bowel is packed away from left hemicolon.

Mobilise: The descending colon is mobilised by division of the peritoneal attachments at the white line of Toldt to the level of the splenic flexure. Great care must be taken to avoid injury to the spleen, also the left ureter, gonadal vessels, kidney, pancreas and fourth part of the duodenum. The transverse colon is mobilised sufficiently to provide a tension-free anastomosis.

Ligation of vessels: Dissection of the mesentery is carried out to identify the inferior mesenteric artery and left colonic branches. These are then isolated, ligated and divided, ensuring that the arterial supply to the proximal and distal margins is not compromised.

Resection of bowel segment: The bowel is clamped and divided, usually with a linear stapling with removal of colonic segment with the associated mesentery.

Restoration of bowel continuity: A handsewn or stapled anastomosis of the descending colon to the rectosigmoid colon is performed. The mesenteric defect is closed to avoid internal herniation. A proximal defunctioning stoma may be fashioned to protect the distal anastomosis.

Closure: Haemostasis is confirmed. A drain is usually placed. Mass closure of the abdominal wall is performed and skin closure is completed with sutures or clips.

COMPLICATIONS

Bleeding, infection, anastomotic leak, ileus, visceral injury, e.g. spleen, herniae, thromboembolism.

Colorectal resection, low anterior

INDICATIONS

Elective: Sigmoid or Rectal tumours, if adequate margins above the anal sphincter complex.

ANATOMY

The rectum (12 cm) begins at the level of the third sacral vertebra, passes downward, lying in the sacrococcygeal curve to the tip of the coccyx. It then bends sharply backward into the anal canal. The mesorectum separates the rectum from presacral (Waldeyer) fascia, hypogastric nerves and autonomic plexus. It contains fatty tissue and lymphatics and total mesorectal excision has been shown to reduce local recurrence rates.

Vascular: The inferior mesenteric artery supplies the upper rectum via the superior rectal artery. The middle and inferior rectal arteries supply the lower rectum and derive from the internal iliac artery. The rectal venous plexus drains into the superior, middle and inferior rectal vessels that are a site of portacaval anastomosis.

Lymphatics: Drainage follows the inferior mesenteric artery to para-aortic nodes.

INVESTIGATIONS

Imaging: CT, MRI scan, endorectal ultrasound: For staging and planning/assessing suitability for anterior resection.

Pre-op: Preoperative chemoradiotherapy may be indicated (reduces local recurrence).

Bowel preparation, bloods: FBC, U&Es, clotting and crossmatch, general anaesthetic assessment and appropriate investigations.

Post-op: Close monitoring. DVT prophylaxis.

PROCEDURE

Position: Patient is positioned in an extended Lloyd-Davis position.

Incision: Lower or extended midline incision or can be performed laparoscopically.

Mobilising the colon: Inspection of the abdominal cavity and assessment of the size and extent of the tumour. The left colon/sigmoid mesentery are mobilised, carefully identifying the ureter and gonadal vessels in the process. The splenic flexure may need to be mobilised.

Mobilising the rectum: The inferior mesenteric artery and vein are dissected, divided and ligated. The sigmoid mesocolon and sigmoid is divided, usually at the apex with a stapler. The rectum can then be retracted forward to further reveal the plane between the mesorectum and the sacral fascia. Dissection continues posteriorly, then laterally around the rectum, producing a characteristic bilobed appearance. The peritoneum is then divided just above the apex of the rectovesical or rectouterine pouch developing the plane between the anterior mesorectum and the seminal vesicles in the male and vagina in female cases.

Resection: Adequate clearance of at least 2 cm is needed proximal and distal to the tumour. Clamps are placed at the distal and proximal resection sites. The lower rectum and anus are washed via proctoscope with antiseptic solution. The bowel is then divided with a stapler between the proximal and the distal clamps.

Anastomosis: Most surgeons use a circular stapling gun. The gun is inserted PR by an assistant and the rod is advanced through the centre of the staple line. The proximal bowel end is sutured around the receiving end of the stapler gun (the anvil). Ensuring no twisting, the stapler is closed and fired which results in a ring of bowel being excised and the two ends being stapled together. The 'donuts' of tissue excised are examined to ensure complete rings and are also sent for histology. The anastomosis can be checked by performing a leak test with air sufflation PR.

Closure: A pelvic drain is usually left *in situ*. The abdominal wall is closed with non-absorbable sutures. Skin closure is completed with sutures or clips. A defunctioning ileostomy is often be fashioned to divert bowel contents while anastomotic healing.

COMPLICATIONS

Bleeding, infection, anastomotic leak, abscess, ileus. Frequency and urgency of bowel motions.

Colorectal resection, right hemicolectomy

INDICATIONS

Elective: Most commonly colonic (caecum, ascending colon or hepatic flexure) or appendiceal neoplasms, e.g. carcinoids >2 cm. Extended right hemicolectomies are performed for tumours involving the hepatic flexure or transverse colon. *Other:* Crohn's disease.

Emergency: Indicated for right colonic obstructing lesions, perforation, haemorrhage or ischaemia, e.g. caecal volvulus or diverticulitis. Ileocaecal resection or limited right hemicolectomy may be necessary in severe appendicitis where the caecum is compromised.

ANATOMY

The ascending colon passes upward from the caecum to hepatic flexure (~15 cm long). It then bends abruptly forward and to the left becoming the transverse colon. The peritoneum covers its anterior surface and sides, i.e. it is retroperitoneal. Important structures to identify and avoid injury during surgery include the right ureter and gonadal vessels, right kidney and duodenum.

Vascular: Arterial supply derives from branches of the superior mesenteric artery, which consists of the right colic, middle colic and ileocolic artery. Venous drainage is variable, mainly via the ileocolic, right colic and middle colic veins into the portal circulation.

INVESTIGATIONS

Imaging: Abdominal radiograph, erect CXR, CT scan: Diagnosis and staging.

Colonoscopy: Diagnosis and biopsy of polyps, tumours, inflammatory bowel, etc.

Pre-op: Bloods: FBC, U&Es, clotting, crossmatch. General anaesthetic assessment and thromboprophylaxis.

Post-op: After elective surgery enhanced recovery: Early return to drinking and eating, early mobilisation, good analgesia, monitor FBC and electrolytes and urine output. If signs of postoperative ileus, then revert to classical nil by mouth ± NG tube and reintroduction of oral liquids then solids as tolerated. Continue thromboprophylaxis.

PROCEDURE

Position: Supine or modified lithotomy.

Access: Midline or transverse incision or laparoscopic approach. Intra-abdominal contents are assessed and the small bowel is packed away.

Mobilise: Lateral to medial or medial to lateral approaches are used. *Lateral to medial:* The lateral peritoneal attachments of the right colon are incised (white line of Toldt) and the hepatic flexure is mobilised by division of the hepatocolic ligament. Careful identification and avoidance of the duodenum, ureter, gonadal vessels. Careful dissection of the correct plane anterior to Gerota's fascia. Dissection of the greater omentum from the area of transverse colon to be divided.

Ligation of vessels: The mesentery from the terminal ileum to transverse colon is dissected carefully to isolate the ileocolic and right colic vessels that are ligated and divided. The right branches of the middle colic artery may also require division.

Resection of bowel segment: Adequate clearance from the lesion is measured and clamps are placed at the two ends of the length to be resected. The bowel is often divided with linear staplers and the right colon is sent for histology.

Restoration of bowel continuity: Bowel ends to be anastomosed should be healthy, well vascularised and tension free. The terminal ileum is anastomosed to the transverse colon in one or two layers using sutures or staples by side-to-side or end-to-end or end-to-side means. The mesenteric defect is closed to prevent internal herniation.

Closure: A drain may be left *in situ*. Following confirmation of haemostasis, mass closure. Skin closure is completed with sutures or clips.

COMPLICATIONS

Anastomotic leak, ileus, abscess, wound infection, thromboembolism, incisional herniae.

Coronary artery bypass graft

INDICATIONS

The main anatomical indications for CABG include:
1. triple coronary vessel disease;
2. left main stem coronary artery disease; and
3. two coronary vessel disease with a proximal left anterior descending artery lesion.

CABG improves long-term survival and relieves angina in these patients.

ANATOMY

The right coronary artery comes off the ascending aorta, runs anteriorly between the pulmonary trunk and the right auricle, and then descends along the atrioventricular groove. At the inferior heart border, it passes posteriorly, anastomosing with the left coronary artery. The left coronary artery arises from the ascending aorta, passes posteriorly between the pulmonary trunk and the left auricle into the atrioventricular groove, dividing into the left anterior descending and the left circumflex arteries. The internal mammary artery, a branch of the subclavian artery, descends along the pleura behind the costal cartilages ending at the sixth intercostal space where it divides to become the superior epigastric and musculophrenic arteries.

INVESTIGATIONS

Pre-op: ECG, echocardiogram, thallium perfusion scintigraphy, coronary angiogram. *Bloods:* FBC, U&Es, clotting and crossmatch. General anaesthetic assessment.

Post-op: Close monitoring in an ITU setting. Rigorous secondary prevention.

PROCEDURE

Incision: Median sternotomy. By incising open and dissecting the pericardium, the heart, coronary vessels and great vessels are exposed and inspected. Minimally invasive thoracotomy incisions are now being performed to reduce the morbidity from sternotomy.

'On pump' CABG: Cardiopulmonary bypass machines, operated by a perfusionist, are used to oxygenate and circulate blood during surgery on the heart. Systemic hypothermia is induced, IV heparin is administered and the venous cannula removes blood from the right atrium, and the blood is returned into the ascending aorta. Cardioplegic solution is administered to the heart to induce a hypothermic, cardioplegic arrest while surgery is performed.

'Off pump' CABG: Instruments called tissue stabilisers are applied to the area of heart where surgery is being performed, allowing the heart to continue beating.

Bypass graft: Arterial grafts include the internal mammary, radial or rarely, gastroepiploic arteries. The internal mammary is mobilised and anastomosed to the coronary artery beyond the stenosis/blockage. Vein grafts are harvested from the long saphenous vein in the leg, through open or minimally invasive incisions and anastomosed from the aorta to the coronary artery beyond the stenosis/blockage.

Closure: The patient is taken off the bypass circuit, allowing the heart to fill and resume contraction. With systemic rewarming, sinus rhythm returns spontaneously or is reinstituted by cardioversion. On satisfactory cardiac output, all cannulas are removed and protamine is administered to reverse heparin. Temporary pacing wires are inserted into the atrium and/or ventricles with two large thoracostomy drains inserted into the pericardium and chest cavity. The sternum is closed with interrupted steel wires and the skin is closed.

COMPLICATIONS

Stroke and neurocognitive dysfunction, intraoperative myocardial infarction, temporary conduction abnormalities and arrhythmias (e.g. atrial fibrillation), pericardial effusion/tamponade, haemorrhage, mediastinitis, sternal wound infection, renal dysfunction, death.

Coronary artery bypass graft (continued)

PROGNOSIS

Operative mortality rate of 2–3.5%. Left internal mammary artery grafts have a 10-year patency of 90%, whereas venous grafts have a 10-year patency of 50–60%. Comparing percutaneous coronary intervention with CABG, the latter has shown a reduced need for revascularisation and a survival advantage for those with diabetes and >65 years.

Endovascular procedures

INDICATIONS

Minimally invasive procedures or 'interventional radiology' for the endoluminal diagnosis and treatment of arterial or venous disorders. Performed by a wide range of specialists including radiologists, vascular surgeons, neurosurgeons, cardiologists and gastroenterologists. Endovascular procedures include:

- Angioplasty and stents for arterial occlusive disease, e.g. coronary, carotid, renal, iliac or limb arteries.
- Stenting of aneurysms, e.g. EVAR and popliteal aneurysms.
- Coil embolisation of aneurysms, e.g. cerebral aneurysms.
- Coil embolisation of bleeding vessels, e.g. gastroduodenal artery in duodenal ulcer bleeding.
- Coil embolisation of dilated veins, e.g. varicocoele and pelvic varicose veins.
- Thrombectomy or catheter-directed thrombolysis.
- Embolisation of tissue, e.g. uterine fibroid embolisation, chemoembolisation of liver metastases.
- Shunts, e.g. transjugular intrahepatic portosystemic shunts (TIPS) in portal hypertension.
- *Filters*: For preventing venous embolism: Inferior vena cava filters.
- *Vein ablation*: Endovenous laser (EVLT) or radiofrequency ablation of varicose veins.

Benefits:

- less pain;
- smaller incisions, often only a puncture wound;
- usually performed under local anaesthesia rather than general anaesthesia;
- lower morbidity and mortality – especially cardiac and pulmonary;
- faster recovery.

PROCEDURE

Access: Local anaesthetic is infiltrated. Percutaneous cannulation and placement of a guidewire and catheter, typically into the femoral artery at the groin for the arterial circulation, femoral vein for venous circulation, under ultrasound guidance. Alternatives include the brachial or axillary, more rarely, subclavian or popliteal arteries. In varicose vein treatment the long saphenous vein is accessed in the lower leg. Antibiotics are administered if device implantation is to be performed.

Navigation: A wide range of types of guidewires and catheters are available. Experience and skill, combined with knowledge of anatomy and imaging enables selective catheterisation of the area of circulation under investigation/treatment. Angiography is performed by injection of radio-opaque contrast to plan, guide and assess therapy.

Angioplasty: Balloon catheters are selected on the basis of the size of the native artery, length of stenosis and lesion distance from access site. After balloon placement across the lesion, the balloon inflation is performed with contrast so that the contour of the balloon can be watched fluoroscopically during dilatation, with measurement of the inflation pressures.

Stents: Can be described as balloon mounted or self-expanding. Many types include bare-metal, drug-eluting and covered stents. Stents used in some areas, e.g. carotid artery, employ embolic protection devices to capture particles of dislodged plaque that embolise and may cause stroke.

Stent graft: Where grafts are supported by a rigid stent structure – used in EVAR.

Coils: These are usually made of platinum, tungsten or nitinol. A delivery wire or 'coil pusher' advances the coil through the microcatheter to the desired intravascular site. The coils are flexible and assume their original shape after deployment blocking further blood flow into the aneurysm or vessel.

Closure: Removal of percutaneous catheter and either manual compression of site or closure devices are used.

Endovascular procedures (continued)

COMPLICATIONS

Site of entry: Haemorrhage, pseudoaneurysm, arteriovenous fistula, groin infection, vessel occlusion.

In the vessel during wire or catheter introduction: False plane, thrombosis, embolism, perforation.

At the site of intervention: Dissection, rethrombosis, intimal flap, perforation, restenosis, stent migration, endoleak, graft infection.

Downstream: Embolisation, thrombosis.

Gastrectomies

INDICATIONS

Elective: Tumours (benign and malignant), severe peptic ulcer disease.

Emergency: Haemorrhage or perforation not controlled by local surgery, gastric necrosis, e.g. secondary to gastric volvulus.

ANATOMY

The stomach can be divided into the cardia, fundus, body, antrum and pylorus, and has lesser and greater curvatures.

Vascular: The arteries supplying the stomach are the left gastric artery, the right gastric artery (usually from hepatic artery), gastroepiploic and short gastric arteries. All of these are branches of the coeliac axis. Venous drainage is into corresponding veins that drain into the portal vein. The gastro-oesophageal junction is a site of portal-systemic anastomosis.

Lymphatics: Lymph nodes are numerous, accompany the arteries and lead to gastric, gastroepiploic, coeliac, portahepatic, splenic, suprapancreatic, pancreaticoduodenal, paraoesophageal and para-aortic lymph nodes.

Nerve supply: *Parasympathetic*: Terminal branches of the right and left vagus nerves. *Sympathetic*: T6–T9 segments passing through the coeliac plexus and distributed through the greater splanchnic nerve.

INVESTIGATIONS

Imaging: *AXR and CXR (erect)*: In an emergency if perforation is suspected. *CT scan:* For staging and assessing resectibility.

Endoscopy: OGD for biopsy, endoscopic ultrasound staging of tumours.

Pre-op: Appropriate bloods: FBC, U&Es, clotting and crossmatch. In gastric tumours, a staging laparoscopy may be performed prior to definitive operation to assess resectibility.

Post-op: NG or nasojejunal tube, urinary catheter, IV fluids. DVT prophylaxis. Parenteral nutrition may be necessary in the immediate post-op period.

PROCEDURE

Incision: *Open*: Usually upper midline or diagonal 'sabreslash' incision. Increasingly performed laparoscopically.

Types of gastrectomies: (See Fig. 23)

- *Billroth I*: Subtotal distal gastrectomy. The proximal stomach lesser curve is reconstructed and then anastomosed to the duodenum. Less commonly performed now.
- *Billroth II (Polya subtotal gastrectomy)*: After resecting the distal stomach, the proximal gastric remnant is anastomosed to the jejunum forming a gastrojejunostomy. The proximal end of the duodenum is oversewn creating a blind loop. With Billroths I and II, there is risk of bile reflux.
- *Roux-en-Y subtotal gastrectomy*: Following resection of the distal stomach, the jejunum is divided with the distal end anastomosed to the gastric remnant, and the proximal jejunum being anastomosed further along the jejunum to form a Roux loop.
- *Total gastrectomy*: The whole stomach is excised and enteric continuity is restored by anastomosing the distal oesophagus to the jejunum, usually by a Roux-en-Y loop.
- *D1 or D2 gastrectomies*: Refers to the radicality of lymph node clearance, D1 involves clearance of N1 or first tier of perigastric nodes, D2 involves more radical nodal clearance (coeliac, splenic, common hepatic nodes). Splenectomy and distal pancreatectomy can be performed, but increases operative mortality (from 4 to 15%) without increasing cancer survival.
- *Two-phase oesophagogastrectomy*: Performed for tumours of the oesophagus or gastro-oesophageal junction. Following abdominal gastric mobilisation and lymphadenectomy, the chest phase involves oesophagectomy, lymphadenectomy, gastric pull up into the chest and formation of a gastric tube conduit.

Gastrectomies (continued)

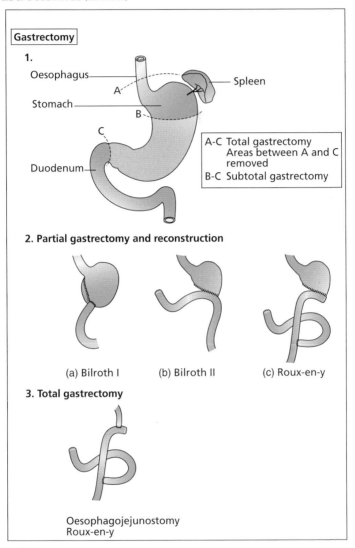

Figure 23 Gastrectomy.

COMPLICATIONS

Early: Bleeding, anastomotic leak, duodenal stump leak, infection, pancreatitis, ileus, fistula formation.

Long-term: Deficiency of Vitamin B_{12}, early and late dumping syndromes, weight loss, reflux, diarrhoea, stomal ulceration, blind loop syndrome, nutritional deficiencies, anaemia, metabolic bone disease.

Laparoscopic abdominal surgery

INDICATIONS

Minimal access surgery of the abdomen or pelvis, whereby following creation of a CO_2 pneumoperitoneum, a laparoscopic camera (either $0°$, $30°$ or $45°$ angle) is introduced into the peritoneal cavity, through a port, for inspection and to guide manipulation of other instruments introduced through other ports.

Diagnostic: Used in the investigation of abdominal or pelvic pain, focal liver disease, abdominal masses, staging of malignant disease, for directed biopsy or emergency evaluation of abdominal trauma.

Therapeutic: Abdominal operations, many procedures can now be carried out by minimal invasive methods. Common procedures include laparoscopic cholecystectomy, appendicectomy, fundoplication, hernia repairs, colectomies, nephrectomy, prostatectomy and bariatric procedures. Laparoscopy can be used to assist in other procedures, e.g. laparoscopic-assisted hysterectomy.

Relative contraindications: Uncorrected coagulopathy, respiratory insufficiency and the presence of distended bowel. Previous open surgery ($\uparrow$ likelihood of adhesions) may make conversion to open more likely.

ANATOMY

Physiological consequences of a pneumoperitoneum are usually well tolerated in otherwise fit patients but may be less so by those with cardiac disease.

Cardiovascular: $\downarrow$ Cardiac output, $\uparrow$ systemic and pulmonary vascular resistance, $\uparrow$ cardiac preload, $\downarrow$ hepatic, splanchnic and renal flow.

Metabolic and autonomic: $\uparrow$ Renin and aldosterone, sympathomimetic response and renal vasoconstriction.

INVESTIGATIONS

Blood: FBC and clotting.

As appropriate for the intended procedure.

PROCEDURE

Performed under general anaesthesia.

Preparation: Nasogastric tube and urinary catheterisation can be used to decompress the stomach and bladder, respectively, depending on the intended procedure. Preparation and draping of the abdomen is performed.

Pneumoperitoneum: Access to the peritoneal cavity can be by three methods:

- *Open (Hassan)*: Following the initial incision, the fascia is exposed. This is divided and fascial sutures can be placed to secure the Hassan trocar. The peritoneum is grasped between two tissue forceps, opened sharply and the Hassan trocar is inserted into the peritoneal cavity under direct vision and insufflation is started.
- *Closed Veress needle*: A Veress needle is introduced into the peritoneal cavity. In the midline, two points of resistance (fascia and peritoneum), more laterally, there are three points of resistance (anterior and posterior sheath and peritoneum). Free flow of saline helps to confirm correct placement. CO_2 insufflation pressures should be low; if high, needle should be repositioned. Once the pneumoperitoneum is established, the needle is withdrawn and a safety shielded trocar is inserted. There is $\uparrow$ risk of damage to bowel or blood vessels as this is a blind procedure.
- *Optical trocar*: A transparent bladeless trocar and a $0°$ laparoscope allows visualisation of the layers of the abdominal wall during direct pressure and twisting to advance the trocar through the abdominal wall. Useful in obese patients.

Insertion of laparoscope: The laparoscope is introduced after adjustment of the white balance (to compensate for the yellow light of the halogen bulb) and used to visualise the peritoneal cavity and safely guide introduction of further ports.

Closure: Following the intended procedure, the instruments and ports are removed under direct vision to ensure no bleeding. Deflation of the pneumoperitoneum and appropriate

Laparoscopic abdominal surgery (continued)

wound closure is performed. In general, 5 mm ports do not need fascial closure, larger ports, e.g. 10–12 mm often need fascial closure, depending on their position, to prevent herniation.

COMPLICATIONS

Immediate: Extraperitoneal insufflation, injury to viscera or vessels (reported incidence of vascular injuries 0.04–0.5%, visceral injuries 0.06–0.12%) with the open Hassan technique having lower incidence than Veress needle or optical trocar. Diaphragmatic splinting due to excessive insufflation. Rarely, pneumothorax or gas embolism.

Early: Shoulder tip pain, wound infection, consequences of unrecognised visceral injury (e.g. peritonitis following bowel injury or consequences of bile duct injury).

Late: Incisional hernia.

Liver resection

INDICATIONS

Elective: Liver tumours: Benign and malignant, primary and secondary.

Indications for colorectal metastases: Solitary or metastases confined to localised area of the liver, with no extrahepatic disease or limited to resectable local recurrence, and hepatic disease can be eradicated with a resection margin of > 5 mm, leaving at least three normal hepatic segments (or more if cirrhosis).

Infections: Occasionally need resection (e.g. hydatid cysts).

Live-related liver donation: Involving partial resection from donor and transplantation of the resected portion into the recipient.

Emergency: Trauma if techniques such as bimanual compression, suture ligation or packing have failed to control bleeding (i.e. resectional debridement of devitalised liver tissue).

ANATOMY

The liver has four lobes, right, left, quadrate and caudate (the latter two anatomically part of the right lobe but functionally part of the left), and is divided into eight segments (of Couinaud), each with their branches of the arterial, venous and biliary systems. They are numbered I to VIII (from left to right). Resections can be segmental or nonsegmental. Normal livers have a great capacity to regenerate, with removal of up to 70% compatible with survival.

Vascular supply: The liver receives 1.5 L blood per minute from the hepatic artery (30%) and the portal vein (70%). Venous flow leads into the three hepatic veins that drain into the inferior vena cava.

INVESTIGATIONS

Patients need to be selected through strict eligibility criteria.

Imaging: CT, MRI, USS may be necessary for staging and planning resections.

Pre-op liver function score: For example, Childs–Pugh scoring (based on bilirubin, albumin, prothrombin time, presence of encephalopathy or ascites): cirrhosis precludes large resections due to the limited reserve of the residual cirrhotic liver.

Blood: FBC, U&Es, clotting and LFT.

Blood products: Blood and FFP should be crossmatched prior to operation as there is high risk of bleeding and transfusion requirement.

PROCEDURE

Should only be carried out in specialist centres with adequate experience.

Incision: Rooftop incision or increasingly performed laparoscopically.

Exploration: Intraoperative ultrasound is used to delineate the borders of a tumour and involvement of surrounding structures (e.g. biliary tree, vessels).

Vascular occlusion: Temporary occlusion of inflow into the liver is achieved either by placing a tourniquet around the portal triad (Pringle's manoeuvre, up to 20 min) or by selective vascular clamping of the Glisson's capsule of the segment.

Liver resection: Parenchymal transaction can be performed by a number of techniques, e.g. harmonic scalpel/ultrasound dissector with meticulous suture ligation or clipping of vessels or ducts. Finally, the resection surface should be carefully inspected for bile leakage or bleeding.

Closure of liver: Resection surfaces can be sealed with either a collagen sponge or a fibrin adhesive.

COMPLICATIONS

Haemorrhage, biliary leakage, liver failure, sepsis (biliary or peritonitis), associated pulmonary complications (e.g. pleural effusion).

Liver transplantation

INDICATIONS

Six hundred to 700 liver transplants are carried out annually in the UK in designated centres with multidisciplinary care.

Elective: For end-stage liver disease (i.e. cirrhosis, with complications such as recurrent variceal haemorrhage, diuretic-resistant ascites, recurrent spontaneous bacterial peritonitis and hepatorenal syndrome). In children, the most common indication is biliary atresia. Organ allocation is on the basis of severity as assessed by the Model for End-Stage Liver Disease (MELD) scoring system (based on bilirubin, creatinine and INR) or Paediatric End-Stage Liver Disease (based on albumin, bilirubin, INR, growth failure and age at listing). The 'Milan criteria' are used in hepatocellular carcinoma: one tumour <5 cm or three lesions <3 cm.

Emergency: Acute liver failure (most common causes are paracetamol overdose, viral hepatitis and idiosyncratic drug reactions).

ANATOMY

Liver transplantation involves the removal of the damaged liver and replacement with a graft in the native hepatic bed, i.e. orthoptic transplantation. The retrohepatic portion of the inferior vena cava is usually removed with the recipient liver, although an alternative technique preserves the recipient's vena cava ('piggyback' technique). In children, splitting of adult donor organs and live-donor segmental (e.g. segments 2 and 3) liver transplantation are performed.

INVESTIGATIONS

Pre-op: Patients undergo a detailed and comprehensive workup prior to placement on the waiting list. This includes a database of liver tests, liver biopsy, blood grouping, tissue typing, ABG, imaging (USS, CT of abdomen, head and chest), ECG and echocardiography, and other assessments, e.g. dental and psychiatry reviews. Once an organ has been allocated, the patient is screened for sepsis (MSU, blood cultures, CXR and ascitic tap).

Post-op: Management is initially on ITU with close monitoring, antibiotics and immunosuppression.

PROCEDURE

Donor organs: Most are from heart-beating donors that have suffered brainstem death. Objective measures of liver status or quality are lacking and, at present, subjective assessment by the surgeon of texture and fat content are used. Live related donors are increasingly being used, e.g. right hemihepatectomy of the donor. Donors and recipients are matched based on blood group and weight.

Organ retrieval: Occurs as part of multi-organ retrieval. The liver is mobilised and the hepatic artery, portal vein, bile duct and supra- and infrahepatic IVC are dissected. Cannulae are inserted into the portal vein and aortic vessels to rapidly infuse the liver with cold preservative solution, e.g. University of Wisconsin solution. The liver is removed with its associated vessels and the biliary system is flushed with preservative solution. Maximum storage time is 15–18 h; with better results, the shorter the preservation period.

Recipient operation: Often technically demanding because of associated portal hypertension and coagulation abnormalities. Close invasive monitoring is required with transfusion of blood products, although this can be reduced by use of a cell saver (collects, washes and recycles RBCs).

Access: A 'Mercedes-Benz incision' is used. The liver is mobilised and vasculature and bile duct is dissected.

Hepatectomy: Recipient hepatectomy involves clamping the IVC and in patients who are unlikely to tolerate the resulting fall in cardiac output, veno-venous bypass is used to divert flow from the IVC, returning via an axillary or jugular vein. *Graft anastomosis:* The donor liver is then anastomosed via the suprahepatic IVC, infrahepatic IVC, portal vein, hepatic artery and then the bile duct by an end-to-end anastomosis or over a T-tube. If the recipient bile duct is diseased, a Roux-en-Y choledochoenterostomy may be performed.

Immunosuppression: Usually a combination of calcineurin inhibitor, e.g. tacrolimus with corticosteroids and an antimetabolite, e.g. mycophenolate mofetil. Monitoring for rejection is carried out by monitoring LFTs and biopsy of the transplanted liver (often via transjugular route).

COMPLICATIONS

Primary graft failure or non-function: <7%, serious complication, requires retransplantation.

Vascular: Haemorrhage, hepatic artery thrombosis, rarely portal vein thrombosis.

Biliary: Bile leakage, later anastomotic stenosis.

Infection: Opportunistic infections, e.g. fungal infections and CMV.

Rejection: Acute: Common, due to T-cells attacking the graft, treated by IV steroid boluses or antibody treatment (antithymocyte globulin).

Chronic (in <5%): Occurs after the first year and is associated with progressive jaundice. Histology shows 'vanishing bile ducts' and small vessel occlusions, usually requires retransplantation.

Recurrent liver disease: Reinfection in the case of hepatitis B or C (if originally present) is common, the latter having the potential for an aggressive and rapidly progressive course. Hepatitis B can be managed with HB-Ig and immunisation. Other diseases that can recur include PBC, PSC and autoimmune hepatitis as well as recidivism in the case of alcoholic liver disease.

Complications of immunosuppression: Drug effects, infections, diabetes, post-transplant malignancies, e.g. skin cancers and lymphomas.

PROGNOSIS

Survival rates are generally good with 85% at 1 year and 70% at 10 years.

Mastectomy

INDICATIONS

Indications for mastectomy in breast cancer include:
- where tumour-free margins cannot be achieved with lumpectomy alone;
- multifocal tumour or widespread carcinoma *in situ*;
- patient preference;
- tumours fixed to underlying muscle, skin or fungating with associated ulceration or bleeding;
- bilateral prophylactic mastectomy, e.g. patients carrying the BRCA-1 or BRCA-2 genes.

ANATOMY

The breast tissue is made up of fatty and glandular tissue (ratio varies from 1:1 to 1:2 in lactation), with a complex network of branching milk ducts that exit on the nipple (from 4 to 18 ducts, the anatomy originally described by Cooper has been radically revised in recent years). The base of the breast covers the second to the sixth rib with an axillary tail. Suspensory connective tissue ligaments extend from the dermis to deep fascia supporting the breast tissue.

Vascular: The breast's arterial supply (and corresponding venous drainage) is from the perforating arteries of the internal mammary and intercostal arteries, also the thoracodorsal, lateral thoracic and thoracoacromial arteries.

Lymphatics: Lymphatics of the lateral half drains into the axillary nodes, comprising anterior, posterior, lateral, central and apical groups, while the medial half drains into the nodes along the internal mammary artery.

INVESTIGATIONS

Pre-op: Tumour diagnosis is based on triple assessment of clinical examination, imaging (mammogram, ultrasound or MRI scan) and cytology/histological analysis by FNA or trucut biopsy. Ideally, a biopsy should confirm carcinoma prior to mastectomy.

Staging investigations: CXR, bone scan, ultrasound, CT and PET scans can be performed. Neoadjuvant chemotherapy may be used to downstage the tumour.

Blood tests: FBC, U&Es, LFT, clotting, G&S or crossmatch. General anaesthetic assessment.

Post-op: DVT prophylaxis, analgesia, physiotherapy to prevent shoulder stiffness, fitting of a bra insert, counseling and support.

PROCEDURE

Total mastectomy	Removal of all breast tissue, overlying skin and the nipple/areola complex
Modified radical mastectomy	Mastectomy with axillary lymph node dissection
Radical or 'Halstead' mastectomy	Mastectomy with axillary lymph node dissection and removal of pectoralis major and minor (no longer performed)
Extended radical mastectomy	Resection of internal mammary lymph nodes
Skin-sparing mastectomy and nipple-sparing mastectomy	Preserves the overlying skin and facilitate immediate reconstruction but are not suitable for tumours near the nipple that are locally advanced or inflammatory in type

Access: An elliptical incision encompassing the lesion and nipple, ensuring wound edges can be approximated.

Modified radical mastectomy: Elevate and dissect skin flaps carefully dividing between subcutaneous and mammary fat avoiding 'button holing'. Dissect superiorly, medially and inferiorly to the limits of breast tissue. Identify the fascia covering pectoralis major and dissect the breast tissue free. If attached, the tumour should be excised with a cuff of muscle. Continue the dissection laterally, to the border of pectoralis major, clearing posteriorly to the anterior border of lattisimus dorsi.

Axillary dissection: The loose areolar tissue of the axilla is dissected with careful identification and preservation of the axillary vessels, thoracodorsal nerve and artery to latissimus dorsi, and long thoracic nerve of Bell that supplies serratus anterior. Nodes removed include the lateral axillary (level I), subscapular, with dissection continued medially for central (level II) and, if necessary, subclavicular nodes (level III), by retraction or division of pectoralis minor, up to the costoclavicular ligament.

Closure: Following confirmation of haemostasis, two drains are inserted, one for the axillary space and the second for the mammary space. The wound is approximated and closed with subcutaneous and skin sutures, avoiding 'dog ears'.

Reconstruction: Mastectomy can be combined with immediate reconstruction by autologous tissue methods, e.g. latissimus dorsi, transverse rectus abdominus or deep inferior epigastric perforator flaps, implant-based methods or a combination of the two. Alternatively, breast reconstruction can be delayed.

COMPLICATIONS

Wound infection, seroma, haemorrhage/haematoma, nerve injury (e.g. long thoracic nerve, thoracodorsal nerve and intercostobrachial nerve), flap necrosis.

Long-term: Poor cosmetic result, lymphoedema to ipsilateral arm, shoulder stiffness, psychological problems, tumour recurrence.

Mastectomy, segmental (wide local excision)

INDICATIONS

Single primary breast tumour that can be excised with clear resection margins (in general <4 cm with 1 cm margins). The patient should be suitable for postoperative radiotherapy and follow-up.

ANATOMY

The breast tissue is made up of fatty and glandular tissue (ratio varies from 1 : 1 to 1 : 2 in lactation), with a complex network of branching milk ducts that exit on the nipple (from 4 to 18 ducts, the anatomy originally described by Cooper has been radically revised in recent years). The base of the breast covers the second to the sixth rib with an axillary tail. Suspensory connective tissue ligaments extend from the dermis to deep fascia supporting the breast tissue.

Vascular: The breast's arterial supply (and corresponding venous drainage) is from the perforating arteries of the internal mammary and intercostal arteries, also the thoracodorsal, lateral thoracic and thoracoacromial arteries.

Lymphatics: Lymphatics of the lateral half drains into the axillary nodes, comprising anterior, posterior, lateral, central and apical groups, while the medial half drains into the nodes along the internal mammary artery.

INVESTIGATIONS

Pre-op: Triple assessment by clinical examination, imaging (ultrasound, mammography or MRI) and cytogical analysis (FNA or trucut biopsy). With smaller, impalpable lesions, imaging-guided wire localisation may be required prior to surgery. *Blood tests:* FBC, U&Es and G&S. CXR and ECG as appropriate. General anaesthetic assessment.

Post-op: DVT prophylaxis. Shoulder exercises to prevent stiffness, especially after axillary surgery.

PROCEDURE

Access: A cosmetically acceptable skin incision should be planned. Options are transverse, circumferential, circumareolar or inframammary. There is usually no excision of skin needed except if required for an adequate tumour-free margin.

Excision: Dissection is performed to remove the breast tissue containing the lesion with adequate margins. The specimen should be marked with sutures to allow accurate orientation for histological analysis. In wire-guided cases, the specimen is X-rayed to ensure complete lesion excision. Breast tissue may need to be mobilised to restore breast shape. Haemostasis should be meticulous.

Closure: Wound is usually closed in two layers, subcutaneous tissue then skin.

Axillary node biopsy, sampling and clearance: Often carried out through a separate incision behind the lateral border of pectoralis major. Sentinal node biopsy is used in patients with clinically uninvolved axilla. Radioactive tracer is injected into the breast in the hours prior to surgery and blue dye (methylene blue) injected at surgery. The first draining nodes are identified and removed for histological analysis. If involved nodes, an axillary clearance is usually performed. The levels of axillary clearance are defined in relation to pectoralis minor, level 1 nodes up to the muscle, level II nodes behind it and level III nodes beyond to subclavius. Careful dissection near the long thoracic nerve of Bell (to serratus anterior), thoracodorsal nerve and vessels (supply latissimus dorsi) and axillary vessels should be performed. The intercostobrachial nerve runs laterally through the axilla and may need to be sacrificed. Following clearance, a drain is usually left *in situ*.

COMPLICATIONS

Bleeding, infection, seroma, poor cosmesis. Of axillary surgery: frozen shoulder, pain, lymphoedema, numbness (intercostobrachial nerve injury), winged scapula (long thoracic nerve injury).

Renal transplantation

INDICATIONS

End-stage renal failure (creatinine clearance <20 ml/min) requiring dialysis or predicted to require dialysis within 6–12 months. Most common causes are diabetic nephropathy, hypertension, glomerulonephritis, reflux nephropathy, polycystic kidney disease and reno-vascular disease.

Renal transplantation is cost-effective when compared to dialysis and also prolongs life expectancy.

ANATOMY

The donor kidney is implanted heterotopically, i.e. in a different location to the native kidney retroperitoneally in the iliac fossa. Renal vessels are anastomosed to the external iliac vessels, or sometimes in children to the aorta and IVC. The ureter is anastomosed to the bladder. Left kidneys are generally less difficult to transplant due to the longer associated vein and artery. Native kidneys are usually left *in situ* unless at risk of causing recurrent sepsis, or in the case of large polycystic kidneys, impinging into the iliac fossa.

INVESTIGATIONS

Preoperative workup: Multidisciplinary assessment including cardiovascular assessment as ischaemic heart disease is very common in patients on dialysis, e.g. ECG, echocardio-graphy, perfusion studies or angiography. Viral screen, e.g. hepatitis B, C, EBV, CMV and HIV.

Living donors: Can be related, non-related or altruistic donors and require a thorough medical and psychological workup. Healthy individuals with normal renal function. Renal vascular anatomy can be investigated with angiography (CT or MR).

Tissue typing and panel-reactive antibody titres: Better matching of major histocompatibility loci class II DR > class I B > class I A results in improved outcome. HLA typing is carried out on patients on the waiting list and also on lymphocytes from the donor lymph node or spleen. Identical or 'favourable' matches are identified, and a national organ-sharing network enables rapid identification of the most suitable recipient. Donor kidneys are blood group compatible and recipients are screened for antibodies that would result in hyperacute rejection. The panel-reactive antibody titre approximates the likelihood that a randomly chosen kidney donor has a positive cytotoxic lymphocyte crossmatch with the potential recipient.

PROCEDURE

Donor organs: Only ~20% of UK patients have suitable living donors; the remainder of organs are from cadaveric donors. Consent from next of kin is obtained in all cases. Donors should have good renal function, be free of systemic infection or malignancy (except for primary brain tumours) and be screened for hepatitis, HIV and CMV status.

Organ retrieval: The kidneys are harvested as part of a multi-organ retrieval, minimising warm ischaemia time, perfusing the kidneys *in situ* with cold preservative solution, e.g. Marshall or University of Wisconsin solution. To avoid damage, the kidney is removed with perinephric fat *in situ*. Preservation times should be minimised but <24 hours is tolerated; any longer can result in higher short- and long-term failure rates. Trials have shown that machine cold perfusion of cadaveric kidneys reduces delayed graft function and improves graft survival.

Recipient operation: An oblique lower abdominal incision is used with an extraperitoneal approach that allows access to the iliac vessels and bladder. The renal vein is anastomosed to the external iliac vein, then usually, an end-to-side arterial anastomosis is created, often with a patch of donor aorta (Carrel patch) (see Fig. 24). A ureteroneocystostomy is then created with a ureteric stent. An indwelling catheter is left for a few days to allow healing of the bladder incision. Antibiotic prophylaxis is given and immunosuppression is commenced. Post-op, careful attention must be placed on fluid balance.

Renal transplantation (continued)

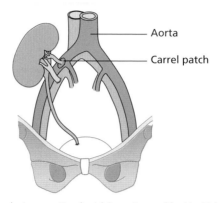

Aorta

Carrel patch

The renal artery on a Carrel patch is anastomosed (end to side) to the external iliac artery. Carrel patch comes from non-living (brain stem dead) donor's aorta

Figure 24 Kidney transplantation.

Immunosuppression: Regimes are based on degree of immunological risk, low or high, e.g. second transplant also risk of diabetes (new-onset diabetes after transplantation, NODAT). Drugs include calcineurin inhibitors, e.g. tacrolimus and cyclosporin; monoclonal antibodies, e.g. basiliximab (IL-2 receptor antagonist); purine synthesis inhibitors, e.g. azathioprine and mycophenolate mofetil, and corticosteroids. Deterioration in renal function is investigated by ultrasound, Doppler and biopsy.

COMPLICATIONS

Impaired graft function: Delayed graft function due to acute tubular necrosis is common (20–30%).

Vascular (1–5%): Haemorrhage, renal artery thrombosis, renal vein thrombosis, renal artery stenosis.

Urological (2–10%): Bladder leak, ureteric leak, ureteric stenosis (treated by ureteroplasty and stent or open surgical intervention) or reflux.

Lymphocoeles: Due to disruption of lymphatics (1–6% of transplants), managed by percutaneous drainage or marsupialisation into peritoneum.

Infection: *Early:* Bacterial infections. *Later:* Opportunistic infections, e.g. CMV, BK virus, HSV, Pneumocystis, Candida.

Rejection:
- *Hyperacute*: Due to preformed antibodies. Pre-transplant crossmatching should prevent this from occurring.
- *Acute*: Most common type (up to 40%). Due to T-cells attacking the graft (diagnosed on derangement of renal function and renal biopsy) and treated by steroid boluses or antibody treatment.
- *Chronic*: Late cause of renal deterioration with gradual reduction of renal function, proteinuria and hypertension. Resistant to most therapies and eventually graft loss will occur.

Immunosuppression: Drug effects, infections, post transplant malignancies, e.g. ↑ risk of skin cancers, lymphomas (post-transplant lymphoproliferative disease).

PROGNOSIS

Patient survival >90% at 1 year, >80% at 5 years. Overall graft survival 85% (cadaveric donor) and 90–95% (living donor) at 12 months with a loss of 3–5% of grafts per year after this. Cardiovascular complications are the most common cause of death post transplant.

Skin grafts and flaps

INDICATIONS

Wounds where primary closure or healing by secondary intention is not possible, would be disfiguring or take a long time, e.g. traumatic skin loss in burns, pressure sores, ulcers, post wide excision after treatment for tumours or infections such as necrotising fasciitis.

Grafts: A skin graft is a piece of skin taken from a donor site and moved to a recipient site. They are free grafts and have to be revascularised from the recipient site. Skin grafts can either be full thickness (Wolfe graft) or split thickness (Thiersch graft). A disadvantage of split skin grafts is their tendency to contract, they are more subject to damage and their cosmetic appearance may be poor. Advantages of full thickness grafts include reduced contraction, ↑ robustness and better appearance, but there is often only a limited area that can be covered and are less reliable than split grafts.

Flaps: A flap is a block of tissue that brings its own blood supply with it. Flaps can be classified on the basis of their blood supply or movement, e.g. advancement or free flaps (the latter involving vascular or microvascular anastomosis), or tissue content, either single (cutaneous, fascial or bone) or composite (myocutaneous or fasciocutaneous). Advantages of flaps are that they can heal many defects and healing times are usually faster than grafts. Disadvantages include the level of expertise required and the donor site may be left with cosmetic or functional defects.

ANATOMY

Partial thickness skin grafts contain epidermis and the superficial part of the dermis skin layers. Epidermis regenerates from the deeper parts of hair follicles and sweat glands. Grafts can be meshed to increase the area that can be covered (creates a 'string vest' appearance), also allows for escape of serous or serosanguinous fluid. Excess skin can be stored aseptically in the fridge for use, ideally <8 days.

Full thickness skin grafts contain the epidermis and dermis. Common donor sites include post-auricular, supraclavicular, lateral groin crease or medial arm. They can only be small size and donor sites are closed primarily or may even require split skin grafting.

INVESTIGATIONS

Pre-op: Recipient wound care, swab to ensure minimal infection. *Streptococcus pyogenes* and *Pseudomonas* should be treated first as they can prevent graft taking. Correct anaemia if significant.

Post-op: Meticulous wound care. Dressings are critical and should not allow the graft to move during bandaging or afterwards or else risk of failure. Assessment of viability or signs of infection.

PROCEDURE

Numerous varied methodologies depending on donor and recipient site.

Split skin grafts: Performed using a Humby knife. Common donor sites are thighs and buttocks. Grafts are anchored at the edges with sutures, staples or glue. Skin grafts take best on granulation tissue; other sites must be sufficiently vascular; tissue such as cartilage, bone or bare tendon will not support a skin graft but may be covered by a skin flap. Following placement, careful dressing is applied to help avoid factors impairing skin graft, including infection, haematoma or seroma and shearing.

Full thickness skin grafts: The pattern of the defect is marked on the donor site and an ellipse cut around the graft to facilitate closure. The graft is then sutured to the recipient site avoiding any tension and carefully dressed.

Skin flaps: Block of skin and underlying tissue (e.g. fascia, muscle or bone) is moved from donor site to a recipient site, bringing its blood supply along. Various techniques are used to move a local flap including advancement, rotation and transposition.

COMPLICATIONS

Infection, haematoma, failure, flap necrosis, scarring, contraction, poor cosmesis.

Splenectomy

INDICATIONS

Traumatic reasons: Rupture after blunt injury to abdomen or iatrogenic during intra-abdominal surgery.

Haematological: Immune thrombocytopaenia, hereditary spherocytosis, elliptocytosis, autoimmune haemolytic anaemias and myelofibrosis; in the past was used for staging of haematological disease, e.g. Hodgkins disease.

Others: Treatment of splenic cysts, tumours, as part of treatment of oesophagogastric varices or splenic artery aneurysms or as part of radical gastrectomies or pancreatectomies.

ANATOMY

The spleen lies posteriorly in the left upper quadrant of the abdomen close to the 9th–11th rib with its long axis lying along the 10th rib. It is surrounded by peritoneum, which passes from hilum to the greater curvature of the stomach and to the left kidney as the gastrosplenic ligament (contains short gastric and left gastroepiploic vessels) and splenorenal ligament (contains splenic vessels and the tail of the pancreas), respectively. It also has avascular ligamentous attachments (e.g. phrenosplenic and splenocolic ligaments).

Main functions: Embryonic haematopoiesis, immunosurveillance: clearance of microorganisms from the blood, formation of immunoglobulin and complement pathway components and removal of senescent red blood cells. Accessory spleens/splenunculi are common (5–15%).

Vascular: The splenic artery is from the coeliac trunk and its venous drainage is via the splenic vein, which runs behind the pancreas, receiving the inferior mesenteric vein, then joins the superior mesenteric vein to form the portal vein.

INVESTIGATIONS

Pre-op: Ideally, vaccination against encapsulated organisms should be given 2 weeks pre-op [Pneumovax (*Streptococcus pneumoniae*), Hib (*Haemophilus influenzae*) and Men C (*Neisseria meningitidis*)]. Appropriate imaging (e.g. CT). FBC, U&Es, clotting and crossmatch. General anaesthetic assessment. Pre-op embolisation may reduce vascularity and aid surgery.

Post-op: Close monitoring. Post-op changes on blood tests include a transient neutrophilia, ↑ number and size of platelets, nucleated red cells and target cells.

Long-term: Patients are prescribed prophylactic antibiotic cover (penicillin V or erythromycin) and lifelong penicillin offered. After emergency splenectomy, vaccination should be given before discharge (may not be as effective if concurrent sepsis). Patients should be given written information and a health alert card. Advice on yearly influenza vaccination.

PROCEDURE

Incision: An upper midline incision for rapid access is used in trauma cases. In elective cases, minimally invasive (laparoscopic) splenectomy is now commonly performed. In the latter, the patient is usually placed in a right-lateral decubitus position with the left arm elevated, allowing the spleen to hang from its diaphragmatic attachments and facilitate dissection.

Open: In trauma cases, the diaphragmatic attachments are divided and the spleen is mobilised medially with packing behind the spleen. The vessels of the splenic hilum are ligated and divided to gain rapid control of bleeding. In non-emergency cases, a more controlled dissection is performed, mobilising the spleen, ligating and dividing the short gastric vessels. Dissection and ligation of the splenic artery and vein near the splenic hilum, taking care not to injury the tail of the pancreas. Careful inspection for haemostasis of the splenic bed. A drain is often placed in the left upper quadrant after surgery. In laparoscopic splenectomy, following dissection, the hilar vessels are ligated with a laparoscopic linear stapler and the spleen is retrieved in a bag through a lower incision, or occasionally fragmented before removal.

COMPLICATIONS

Short-term: Haemorrhage, gastric dilatation, pancreatic fistula, infection – subphrenic collection or abscess.

Long-term: ↑ Risk of sepsis, especially encapsulated organisms, overwhelming post-splenectomy infection (OPSI). Increased risk of malaria in travel to endemic areas.

Stomas

INDICATIONS

A surgically created opening of the bowel or urinary tract to a body surface. Commonest types of stomas are ileostomy, colostomy and urostomy (others include oesophagostomy, gastrostomy, jejunostomy and caecostomy). Can be permanent or temporary, end or loop stomas.

Elective: In inflammatory bowel disease, malignancy. End ileostomies after a panproctocolectomy for ulcerative colitis or familial polyposis. Permanent colostomies after abdominoperineal resection for low rectal carcinomas. Loop stomas used to temporarily divert bowel contents to protect distal surgery, e.g. an ileoanal pouch or low colorectal anastomosis, anal sphincter repair or to divert bowel content from diseased segments of bowel.

Emergency: Bowel trauma, perforation, obstruction, ischaemia, inflammatory bowel disease, e.g. toxic megacolon. In a Hartmann's procedure, the diseased distal colon is resected with formation of an end colostomy and the distal end of the divided bowel is closed or formed into a mucous fistula.

ANATOMY

End stoma: The bowel is divided and the proximal end is brought through the abdominal wall to form the stoma. The distal end can be closed and left in the abdomen, brought out through a separate incision (mucous fistula) or in the same opening to form a double-barrel stoma (see Fig. 25).

Loop stomas: A loop of bowel is brought up to the surface, opened and folded back on itself to form a stoma with two lumens. Can be easier to close. Some risk of 'spillover' of proximal contents.

Ileostomies: Often, but not always, situated in the right iliac fossa. As output is irritant, they are formed with a spout, projecting ~2.5 cm above the skin surface. Output is liquid and about 1–2 L/day, although it may diminish after a few weeks.

Colostomies: Often sited in the LIF although maybe anywhere, with the stoma flush to the skin. Output is intermittent and of a more solid consistency, depending on diet (although transverse colostomies have a more frequent semi-liquid output and can be more difficult to manage).

Stoma appliances: Consist of a pouch and a flange (the portion that sticks to and protects the skin around the stoma). The flange may consist of one or two pieces, the second piece being left attached to the skin for a few days when the pouch is changed. Some bags also have exit drains (e.g. for ileostomies) for liquid output. Charcoal filters can be used to reduce odour of flatus.

INVESTIGATIONS

Pre-op: Although not always possible in emergency situations, stoma siting and counselling is important. Stoma care nurse specialists are vital. Stomas should be marked pre-op, where the patient can see the stoma, avoiding skinfolds, scars, bony prominences and the belt line. Bowel preparation may be required. Prior to stoma reversal, distal contrast studies are often required.

Post-op: DVT prophylaxis. Patient education and support for managing stoma.

PROCEDURE

Skin incision: A circular skin opening is created at the site marked for the stoma (placing a stoma through the rectus muscle minimises the chance of developing a parastomal hernia). The skin is incised, fascia divided, the muscle split and the peritoneum is opened (should accommodate two fingers). *Stoma formation:* The end or loop of bowel is brought out through the opening. This should be tension free, untraumatised and well-vascularised bowel. The main incision is closed and dressed. The bowel is opened if it has previously been stapled or is a loop and the edges are cleaned. The bowel is everted on itself and the edges sutured to the skin. A transparent stoma bag is then applied to allow regular stoma inspection.

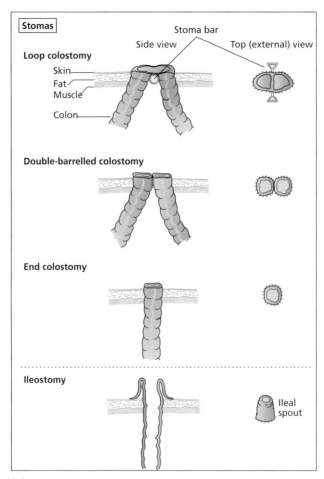

Figure 25 Stomas.

Relatively common (40% for ileostomies and 20% for colostomies), with ~15% necessitating operative correction.

Necrosis: Becomes evident within a few hours of surgery, due to compromise of the blood supply to the bowel during stoma formation, requires revision of stoma.

Haemorrhage: A minor degree is common and rarely requires intervention.

Functional: Diarrhoea or constipation. Output from ileostomies can be of large volume liquid resulting in dehydration and electrolyte imbalances (can be managed by fluid replacement and medications, e.g. loperamide and codeine). Urinary tract calculi are more common in individuals with an ileostomy; hence the importance of hydration.

Other: Skin irritation, leakage, prolapse or retraction, occasionally requiring refashioning, stenosis (may be possible to dilate using a dilator), otherwise refashioning, parastomal hernias, abscess or fistula.

Psychological: Embarrassment, anxiety or body image problems.

Suturing

INDICATIONS

Wounds or surgical cuts requiring closure. The aim is to appose wound edges without tension to enable rapid healing with good cosmesis.

ANATOMY

The skin is divided into three layers:
(1) **epidermis** – outer keratinised epithelium;
(2) **dermis** – underlying fibroelastic layer containing blood vessels, lymphatics and nerves;
(3) **subcutaneous tissue** – deep layer of variable thickness comprising mostly adipose tissue.

INVESTIGATIONS

Pre-op: Informed consent, history of allergy to skin prep or antibiotics. Appropriate lavage and toilet of traumatic wounds. It is always important to consider tetanus status and give booster or immunoglobulin and immunisation as appropriate. Radiographs may be necessary if there is risk of foreign body such as glass or associated bony injury.

Post-op: Wound care advice, analgesia, dressings and antibiotics only if appropriate.

PROCEDURE

Simple lacerations may be closed primarily. More complex injuries, especially involving face or other injuries, e.g. tendon damage, are best referred to appropriate specialists, e.g. plastic surgeons. If associated with a fracture, i.e. an open fracture, antibiotics should be given. For cuts caused by bites, primary closure is avoided and antibiotics given, especially in human bites.

Local anaesthesia: Following skin preparation, local anaesthetic is infiltrated around the wound, ensuring aspiration prior to injection to avoid intravascular injection. Local anaesthetic mixed with adrenaline should never be injected near digits or areas such as nose, ear or penis.

Inspection and wound toilet: The wound is inspected and thoroughly irrigated and cleaned. This may require scrubbing if dirty. The wound is inspected for any underlying damage, e.g. to tendons.

Type of suture: Sutures can be classified as absorbable or non-absorbable, monofilament or multifilament (braided), natural or synthetic. If deep tissues require suturing, subcutaneous absorbable sutures are used. Otherwise non-absorbable sutures are always used in traumatic wounds. This allows an individual or limited number to be removed if infection develops without compromising the whole wound. Absorbable sutures are often used in surgical wounds. Suture width used depends on site, e.g. finer 5–0 or 6–0 sutures for face, 3–0 or 4–0 for trunk/arms and 2–0 for scalp.

Suturing: See Fig. 26 for a diagrammatic summary of types. Aseptic technique should be used with appropriate wound preparation and draping. Simple discontinuous (interrupted) sutures are commonly used. Vertical mattress stitches may be used for deeper wounds; they enable good skin edge eversion. Subcuticular suturing enables close wound approximation, with good cosmesis.

Dressing: A dry dressing is applied to the wound. Stitches are kept in place only as long as needed to provide support to the wound. Stitches on the face are removed within 2–5 days, whereas limb and abdominal wall stitches usually remain for 7–10 days.

COMPLICATIONS

Poor cosmesis, sutures can act as nidus for infection, stitch abscess, stitch granuloma, stitch sinus, wound dehiscence, scarring.

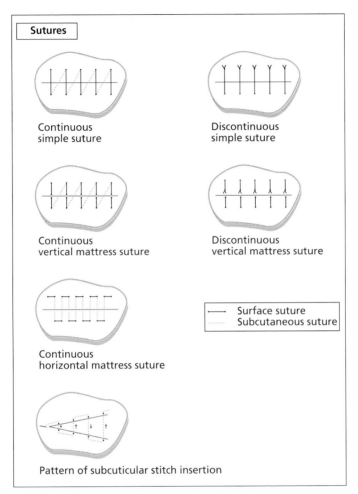

Figure 26 Skin suturing techniques.

Thyroidectomy

INDICATIONS

Benign and malignant thyroid tumours; definitive diagnosis of thyroid mass when FNA equivocal. Symptomatic goiters (pressure effects or cosmesis). As therapy for thyrotoxicosis, Graves' disease or toxic nodular goitre.

ANATOMY

The thyroid gland consists of two lobes connected by the thyroid isthmus that overlies the second and third tracheal rings. The gland is enclosed in the pretracheal fascia, lies deep to the strap muscles.

Vascular: The gland is supplied by the superior thyroid artery from the external carotid, the inferior thyroid artery from the thyrocervical trunk of the subclavian and sometimes the thyroidea ima artery from the aortic arch or brachiocephalic artery. Venous drainage is via the superior, middle and inferior thyroid veins into the internal jugular vein.

INVESTIGATIONS

Bloods: Thyroid function tests – patients with hypo- or hyperthyroidism should treated medically preoperatively, full blood count, renal function and calcium.

Ultrasound: To define a lesion or assess a goitre. CT scan to assess retrosternal extension and tracheal narrowing. Nuclear medicine scintigraphy if appropriate.

Ultrasound-guided FNA or biopsy: For cytological diagnosis.

Indirect laryngoscopy: To assess vocal cord function preoperatively.

Post-op: Monitoring and replacement of calcium if required. Thyroxine replacement.

PROCEDURE

Positioning: Reverse Trendelenburg, head up with neck extended.

Incision: Skin crease collar incision two fingerbreaths above the suprasternal notch. Subcutaneous tissue and platysma are divided and flaps are elevated superiorly to the thyroid cartilage and inferiorly to the sternum avoiding injury to the anterior jugular veins.

Thyroid exposure and mobilisation: A Jolls' retractor is used to retract the subplatysma flaps. The strap muscles are separated by dividing up the midline raphe to expose the thyroid gland underneath. The thyroid gland is exposed. Middle thyroid vein(s) are carefully ligated, looking for and avoiding the parathyroids (small tan glands). The superior pole vessels are dissected, clipped away from the gland, divided and doubly ligated. The recurrent laryngeal nerve runs in the tracheooesophageal groove and should be carefully identified and preserved, avoiding diathermy near the nerve. Although usually deep to the lower pole vessels, it can run between or infront. The inferior thyroid vascular pedicle is carefully ligated near the thyroid. If hemithyroidectomy, the isthmus is oversewn with absorbable sutures.

Closure: Good haemostasis is essential. Many surgeons will leave a vacuum drain in situ. Closure is in three layers, opposition of the strap muscles, subcutaneous tissue, platysma and skin.

COMPLICATIONS

Bleeding, breathing difficulties caused by haematoma compressing the trachea or bilateral recurrent laryngeal nerve damage, voice changes – recurrent laryngeal nerve damage, hypocalcaemia, hypothyroidism, wound infection.

Tracheostomy

INDICATIONS

Most common indication is longer term ventilatory support (or weaning), others include trauma, neurological impairment (e.g. coma, stroke and motor neurone disease), head and neck surgery and bilateral vocal cord paralysis.

ANATOMY

The trachea made up of semicircular cartilage rings, incomplete posteriorly (membranous part). The anterior surface of the trachea is convex, and covered (superiorly to inferiorly), by the isthmus of the thyroid gland (over second and third rings), the inferior thyroid veins, the strap muscles of the neck and the cervical fascia. The recurrent laryngeal nerves and the inferior thyroid veins lie in the tracheooesophageal grooves laterally and can be vulnerable to injury.

Types of tracheostomy: Can be plastic, silicone or metal, cuffed or uncuffed, or fenestrated (allows speech as tube has a hole that allows air through the upper airway when the external opening is blocked). Most have an outer cannula, an inner cannula and an obdurator that guides insertion but is removed once in place.

INVESTIGATIONS

Performed under general anaesthesia.

Pre-procedure: When possible, pre-procedure counselling on risks, benefits is recommended.

Post-procedure: Close care is important. Humidified gases and regular sterile suction of retained secretions. Cuffed tracheal tubes allow positive pressure ventilation but pressure should be monitored and deflated regularly to prevent pressure necrosis. After 5–7 days, the tracheostomy tube can be replaced.

PROCEDURE

Access: The patient is positioned with the neck extended. A vertical or transverse incision is made midway between sternal notch and cricoid cartilage. To expose the trachea, dissect through subcutaneous tissue and platysma, split and retract the strap muscles and, if necessary, divide the thyroid isthmus.

Surgical tracheostomy: Make a longitudinal or U-shaped incision in the trachea (two to three tracheal rings in length). Stay sutures can be placed laterally to help hold the trachea open and left in situ for ease of replacement should the tracheostomy tube be dislodged. Insert a tracheostomy tube (it may be necessary to remove the endotracheal tube at the same time). Inflate the balloon of the tracheostomy tube and secure in place with sutures to the skin.

Percutaneous tracheostomy: Can be performed in ITU/HDU settings. Uses a bronchoscope and a Seldinger technique to cannulate the trachea percutaneously, placement of a guidewire and progressive dilators before placement of tracheostomy tube. Not suitable for patients with difficult anatomy, obesity, coagulopathy or thyroid enlargement.

COMPLICATIONS

Short-term: Bleeding, infection, pneumothorax or pneumomediastinum, subcutaneous emphysema, injury to adjacent structures, e.g. recurrent laryngeal nerves, oesophagus, vessels, tube displacement, tracheal ulceration, tracheitis, mucus plugging, aspiration.

Long-term: Tracheal stenosis, tracheomalacia, overgranulation, tracheo-oesophageal fistula (<1%), persistent tracheocutaneous fistula.

Vascular access

INDICATIONS

Access for haemodialysis: Involves creation of a fistula 2–3 months before dialysis is due to begin. Ideally, a native fistula, as distally as possible to provide optimal length for vein cannulation and allow later creation of more proximal access if fails, also limits chance of cardiac strain and 'steal syndrome'.

Indications for leg fistula: Innominate vein or superior vena cava occlusion (most commonly due to previous central vein lines).

Indications for graft fistula: Exhausted peripheral veins, central vein occlusion or severe obesity.

Central vein catheters: Required if a patient needs urgent haemodialysis and no working fistula, severe heart failure or peripheral vascular disease.

ANATOMY

Three main options: native arteriovenous fistula (AVF), prosthetic arteriovenous graft (AVG) or central venous catheter.

Native fistulas: Radiocephalic (Brescia–Cimino), more proximal radiocephalic fistula, brachiocephalic, brachiobasilic, atypical (ulnarbasilic or radiobasilic), upper leg: saphenous vein loop, saphenous vein in situ, femoral vein loop.

Complex vascular access procedures: Axillary artery to contralateral axillary vein (necklace graft), axillary loop graft and contralateral IJV bypass graft. Femoro-femoral crossover bypass, SFV transposition (SVC obstruction) and axillary artery-popliteal vein bypass graft (SVC obstruction in diabetic or obese patients).

Central venous catheters: Non-tunnelled (short-term) or tunnelled (cuffed to prevent infection) catheters, single lumen and double lumen.

INVESTIGATIONS

Pre-op: Careful clinical assessment of arterial and venous anatomy. Allen test. If indicated, e.g. history of vascular problems or difficulty in assessment, duplex scanning to assess arterial inflow, vein caliber and patency. Venogram if there is question over venous patency.

Post-op: Assessment of fistula with clinical examination of thrill, bruit. Native fistulae need time to mature, usually a few weeks, before they can be used for dialysis. Grafts can be needled more quickly.

Follow-up care: Ultrasound dilution assessment to measure graft inflow rate, recirculation rate and cardiac output. If inflow <600 ml/min, a fall since previous examination, or recirculation rate >5%, a fistulogram can be performed and appropriate intervention performed, e.g. fistuloplasty of stenosis (endovascular or surgical).

Anaesthesia: Local, regional block or general anaesthesia depending on surgery.

PROCEDURE

Following an appropriate incision, the vein is assessed, dissected, mobilised and divided distally. The artery is dissected and following IV administration of heparin, clamped and an arteriotomy is made. An end to side anastomosis is performed with prolene suture. In brachiobasilic fistulae, the vein has to be transposed into superficial subcutaneous tissue to allow easy cannulation. Grafts used are usually PTFE, straight or looped.

Central venous catheters: Placement under ultrasound guidance, usually internal jugular vein, the femoral vein can be used but only short term due to the risk of infection and thrombosis.

COMPLICATIONS

Bleeding, infection, nerve injury, distal embolisation, steal syndrome, thrombosis, failure to mature, stenosis, cardiac strain, limb swelling, aneurysmal dilatation.

Vasectomy

INDICATIONS

Elective: contraception (should be considered irreversible). Rarely, recurrent epididymitis ($\downarrow$ risk by 60%).

ANATOMY

The vas deferens (ductus deferens) is a duct that delivers spermatozoa produced in the testes, from the tail of the epididymis to the ejaculatory ducts. It is 45 cm long and traverses the scrotum and the inguinal canal. It crosses the external iliac artery, entering the pelvis below the peritoneum covering the lateral wall. At the ischial tuberosity, it turns medially and crosses in front of the ureter to the base of the bladder where it joins the ipsilateral seminal vesicle to form the ejaculatory duct that travels through the prostate gland to open into the prostatic urethra.

Vascular: The artery to the vas is from the internal iliac artery and may be encapsulated by venous varicosities, i.e. varicocele in the scrotum.

INVESTIGATIONS

Pre-op: Patient and partner should be counselled, informed consent. It should be stressed to the patient that this procedure should be considered irreversible. Medical history is reviewed and certain medication stopped, e.g. aspirin 1 week pre-op if appropriate.

Post-op: Scrotal support is worn for up to 1 week. Patient should be warned to continue using pre-op contraceptive methods for $\sim$12 weeks and two separate semen samples should confirm azoospermia.

PROCEDURE

Performed under local anaesthesia. Skin should be shaved and cleaned with antiseptic. The two main techniques are scalpel and no-scalpel:

Scalpel: The vas deferens is held between the thumb and two fingers, and local anaesthetic is infiltrated, usually at the junction of the middle and upper one-third of the scrotum bilaterally. A small vertical incision is made over the vas on the scrotal surface. Surrounding tissue is bluntly dissected away, the vas deferens drawn out of the incision and a clip used to grasp the midportion. The vas is ligated and a length excised (usually $\sim$1–2 cm). Cauterisation to the cut ends, folding back the vas or fascial interposition is used to prevent recanalisation. Haemostasis should be meticulous. Skin closure is achieved with simple interrupted sutures. This is repeated on the other side.

No-scalpel: The vas deferens is palpated under the skin and clamped with a ring forceps. Skin is pierced with a dissecting forceps and used to create an opening. The vas is drawn out with the ring clamp and treated as with the scalpel technique.

The excised segment of the vas should be sent for histological confirmation.

COMPLICATIONS

Short-term: Infection, bruising, bleeding/haematoma, sperm granuloma, epididymitis.

Long-term: Less than 1% failure rate (i.e. conception) due to recanalisation, surgical error, anatomical variants or failure of contraception prior to confirmation of azoospermia. Scrotal pain is uncommon.

Whipple's procedure (pancreatoduodenectomy)

INDICATIONS

Tumours of head of pancreas, duodenum, ampulla or distal common bile duct (in general, <20% patients have disease that is resectable).

ANATOMY

The pancreas is a retroperitoneal structure in the transpyloric plane. The four parts are the head, neck, body and tail. The head lies in the curve of the duodenum. A Whipple's procedure involves *en bloc* removal of the distal stomach (except in pylorus preserving pancreatectomy), duodenum, head of the pancreas, distal common bile duct and gallbladder (see Fig. 27). Enteric continuity by the formation of a pancreaticojejunostomy, choledochojejunostomy and gastrojejunostomy More recently, pylorus-preserving pancreaticoduodenectomy has been shown to improve gastrointestinal function, as indicated by improved weight gain, less ulceration and dumping syndrome.

Vascular: Blood supply to the pancreas is from the splenic and pancreaticoduodenal arteries. Venous drainage is via the splenic and pancreaticoduodenal veins to the portal vein.

INVESTIGATIONS

Endoscopy ± ERCP: diagnosis and histology.

Imaging: CT, MRCP, endoscopic ultrasound, angiography and FDG-PET scanning: diagnosis, staging and assessment of resectability.

Blood: FBC, U&E, LFT, CA19-9 and CEA.

Pre-op: Multi-disciplinary discussion, blood and crossmatch, biliary decompression or stenting may be required. Cover with broad-spectrum antibiotics.

Post-op: ITU/HDU care and close monitoring, insulin for blood glucose control, H2 receptor antagonists or proton pump inhibitors, octreotide and thrombo-prophylaxis, long term: pancreatic enzyme supplementation. Adjuvant chemoradiotherapy may be indicated.

PROCEDURE

Positioning: Supine.

Incision: Roof top, vertical midline or transverse can be used.

Inspection: Abdominal contents and lesion inspected for resectability. If unresectable, then palliation by bypass, e.g. gastrojejunostomy and choledocho- or cholecystojejunostomy.

Mobilisation: The duodenum is mobilised (Kocherisation) and the distal stomach divided or the duodenum divided 2 cm distal to the pylorus in pylorus-preserving procedure. The duodenum is resected together with the gallbladder, common bile duct, proximal pancreas with lymph node dissection. Frozen section can be used to ensure clear margins on pancreatic resection. End-to-side or end-to-end pancreaticojejunostomy is performed. Further downstream, an end-to-side hepaticojejunostomy and end-to-side gastrojejunostomy or pylorus-jejunotomy is made. A feeding jejunostomy can be fashioned for nutritional support.

Closure: Careful heamostasis. Placement of drains. Mass closure. Skin may be closed with subcuticular suture or clips.

COMPLICATIONS

Morbidity is high (40%). Bleeding, anastomotic leak, biliary leak, ileus, diabetes, abdominal or wound sepsis, delayed gastric emptying, pancreatitis, pancreatic fistula, pancreatic insufficiency, weight loss, dumping and reflux.

PROGNOSIS

A major surgical procedure that should be performed in specialist centres where mortality rates are now <5%. Resectable tumours 30% 5-year survival.

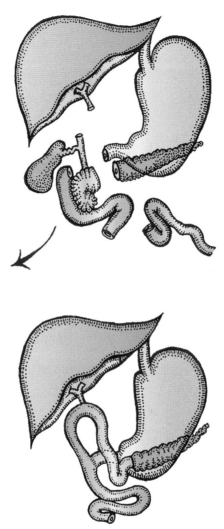

Figure 27 Whipples pylorus preserving pancreaticoduodenectomy. (Top) Removal of the duodenum, head of the pancreas, distal common bile duct and gallbladder. (Bottom) Reconstruction after
resection.

Achalasia

DEFINITION
A motor disorder of the oesophagus with failure of lower oesophageal sphincter (LES) relaxation and loss of peristalsis on swallowing.

AETIOLOGY
Degeneration of intramural ganglions of myenteric (Auerbach's) plexus causes impaired relaxation of the lower sphincter and disrupts peristaltic coordination. Cause of the degeneration is unknown and may be autoimmune or infective. *Trypanosome cruzi*, a parasitic protozoon, can cause a similar syndrome, but this is confined to South America.

EPIDEMIOLOGY
Incidence of 0.5/100,000 per year. Predominantly in middle ages. No racial or gender differences.

HISTORY
Dysphagia, initially intermittent, involving solids and liquids. Undigested food or retained saliva may be regurgitated (particularly at night); atypical/cramping retrosternal chest discomfort or fullness, coughing/recurrent chest infection and weight loss are common.

EXAMINATION
No signs. There may be evidence of complications.

INVESTIGATIONS
Barium swallow: Absent peristalsis in the body of oesophagus that smoothly tapers down to the lower oesophageal sphincter 'bird's beak' appearance. Tortuous dilated oesophagus with retained food in long-standing disease (where CXR may show dilated oesophagus, double right heart border and fluid level behind heart shadow (see Fig. 28)).

Oesophagoscopy/endoscopic ultrasound: To exclude malignancy (tumour may cause pseudoachalasia) or stricture. Biopsy not necessary for diagnosis but may show muscle hypertrophy/lack of nerve fibres.

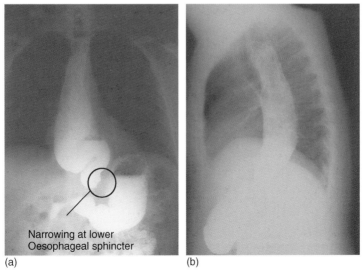

Narrowing at lower
Oesophageal sphincter

(a)   (b)

Figure 28 Barium swallow demonstrating failure of relaxation of LES with proximally dilated oesophagus (a) AP view (b) lateral view.

Achalasia (continued)

Oesophageal manometry: Classical findings are: elevated lower oesophageal sphincter pressure, failure of lower oesophageal sphincter to relax on swallowing and aperistalsis of oesophageal body. 'Vigorous' achalasia: where patients have high-amplitude peristaltic contractions of the body of the oesophagus on swallowing with associated pain.

Blood: Exclusion of Chagas' disease (serology against *T. cruzi*) is rarely necessary.

MANAGEMENT

All treatment options aim to reduce the lower oesophageal sphincter pressure:

Medical: Nifedipine or verapamil (calcium channel antagonists) or isosorbide mononitrate pre-meals (short-term relief).

Endoscopic: Pneumatic balloon dilatation of LES (80% success rate, but small risk of perforation). Botulinum toxin injection into the LES is effective in >75% of patients; however, symptoms recur within 6 months, serial treatments are required and there may be a decline in response. Usually limited to patients unsuitable for balloon dilatation or surgery.

Surgery: Heller's cardiomyotomy: anterior myotomy of LES is now mostly performed laparoscopically (a robotic approach is performed in some centres). Heller's cardio-myotomy can be combined with fundoplication (usually anterior Dor) to prevent gastro-oesophageal reflux. Results: good-to-excellent relief of symptoms.

COMPLICATIONS

If untreated, aspiration pneumonia, malnutrition and weight loss may result. In time, there is increased risk of oesophageal malignancy, especially squamous cell carcinoma, and endoscopic surveillance and biopsy is recommended.

Of Heller's: Perforation (7–15%), increased risk in patients who have had previous Botox injection due to submucosal fibrosis, reflux, and recurrence (early: technical failure or scarring, late: disease progression).

PROGNOSIS

No cure but up to 90% of patients can be managed effectively with single or multiple treatment modalities.

Gastric cancer

DEFINITION
Gastric cancer, most commonly adenocarcinoma, more rarely lymphoma, leiomyosarcoma.

AETIOLOGY
Associated with *Helicobacter pylori* infection and atrophic gastritis.
Germline mutations in E-cadherin in hereditary diffuse gastric cancer.
Diet high in smoked and processed foods, nitrosamines, smoking, alcohol.
Blood group A (1.2 × relative risk).
Pernicious anaemia.
Previous partial gastrectomy.
MALT lymphomas are very strongly causally associated with *H. pylori* infection.

EPIDEMIOLOGY
Common cause of cancer death worldwide, with highest incidence in Japan, China, Eastern Europe. Sixth commonest cancer in the UK (incidence is 15/100,000). Male:female is ~2 : 1. Usual age of presentation >50 years. Cancer of the antrum/body is decreasing, while that of the cardia and gastro-oesophageal junction is increasing.

HISTORY
Early asymptomatic; later, early satiety, anorexia, nausea, epigastric pain/indigestion anaemia/GI bleeding and weight loss. Symptoms of metastatic disease: abdominal distention (ascites), jaundice (liver involvement).

EXAMINATION
Late signs: Epigastric mass, ascites.
Eponymous signs found in metastatic spread:
- *Virchow's node or Troisier's sign*: Palpable lymph node(s) in the left supraclavicular fossa.
- *Sister Mary Joseph's node*: Metastatic nodule on umbilicus.
- *Krukenberg tumour*: Metastases to ovary.

INVESTIGATIONS
Upper GI endoscopy: With multi-quadrant biopsy of all gastric ulcers.
Endoscopic ultrasound: Assess depth of gastric invasion (T stage) and local lymph node involvement.
CT scan: Staging of tumour.
Staging laparoscopy: Enables examination for local or transperitoneal spread.
Pathology: Macroscopic: Polypoid, ulcerating or infiltrative tumours (Borrmann's classification); if widespread, may cause linitis plastica (leather-bottle stomach). Microscopic: Intestinal and diffuse types.

MANAGEMENT
Surgery: Mainstay for early disease – subtotal or total gastrectomy (see Gastrectomies). Lymph node dissection termed D1 (including perigastric N1 nodes), and D2 (with N2 tier of nodes) (Japanese proponents for the latter). Increased morbidity and mortality in total and D2 gastrectomy. At least 15 nodes required for staging.
Palliative: For example, gastrojejunostomy or stenting to maintain enteral nutrition.
Medical: Neoadjuvant chemotherapy has been shown to improve survival (MAGIC trial, ECF chemotherapy, 36% versus 23% for surgery alone 5-year survival). Advanced disease: Therapy is aimed at palliation. Higher response rates in combination chemotherapy.

COMPLICATIONS
Upper GI haemorrhage, iron deficiency anaemia, dysphagia, gastric outlet obstruction. Early and late complications of gastrectomy (e.g. dumping syndrome, diarrhoea, deficiencies of vitamin B_{12}).

Gastric cancer (continued)

Gastric carcinomas can spread directly through stomach wall, via lymph nodes, transperitoneal or haematogenous to liver, lungs.

PROGNOSIS

Generally poor with ~20% overall 5-year survival (60% in Japan), higher in those with early disease undergoing resection.

Staging: TNM system or the Birmingham Staging System based on clinical and pathological data.

Gastrointestinal haemorrhage, upper

DEFINITION

Haemorrhage arising from the upper part of the gastrointestinal tract, i.e. proximal to the ligament of Treitz.

AETIOLOGY

Acute or chronic: Gastric and duodenal ulcer (50% of cases), acute erosive gastritis, oesophagitis or duodenitis, oesophageal or gastric varices, Mallory–Weiss tear, gastric angiodysplasia or Dieulafoy's malformation, tumours or rarely haemobilia, aorto-enteric fistula or amyloidosis.

ASSOCIATIONS/RISK FACTORS

Helicobacter pylori, NSAIDs and steroids are risk factors for the development or exacerbation of ulcers and erosions. Stress ulcers 2° to shock and ↓ splanchnic perfusion (Curling's ulcers in burns, Cushing's ulcer in head injury). Alcoholic binges can precipitate gastric erosions. Repeated vomiting ↑ risk of a Mallory–Weiss tear.

EPIDEMIOLOGY

A common emergency presentation, 50–80/100,000 upper GI bleeds annually in the UK. More common in older individuals.

HISTORY

History suggestive of cause (e.g. alcoholism, NSAID use, vomiting).

Acute: Haematemesis of fresh blood or dark, partly digested blood ('coffee grounds'), melaena (loose black tarry offensive stools), suggesting a bleed of >50 mL or, if rapid bleeding, frank PR blood loss.

Chronic: Iron deficiency anaemia, positive faecal occult blood.

EXAMINATION

Signs of iron deficiency anaemia (chronic) or other signs, e.g. palmar erythema, spider naevi, bruising, ascites or jaundice in liver disease, orofacial telangiectasia in Osler–Weber–Rendu syndrome.

Signs of shock, hypotension, tachycardia, hypovolaemia, altered mental status.

INVESTIGATIONS

Blood: FBC, U&Es, clotting, LFT, crossmatch.

Oesophagogastroduodenoscopy (OGD): Identifies site of bleeding and allows treatment. Stigmata of recent haemorrhage include active bleeding, visible vessel or adherent clot. Posterior duodenal ulcers can erode and cause massive bleeding from the gastroduodenal artery.

Mesenteric angiography: Localises source of bleeding, but rates must be 1–1.5 mL/minute, allows treatment by embolisation.

MANAGEMENT

Resuscitation: ABCs, adequate IV access, active resuscitation with fluid/blood products and correction of coagulopathy.

Medical: PPI or H2-antagonist to reduce acid secretion. *H. pylori* eradication once stable in duodenal ulceration. Vasopressin or somatostatin analogues (e.g. octreotide) reduce splanchnic blood flow and portal pressure and are useful in variceal bleeding. A Sengstaken–Blakemore tube can be inserted for mechanical compression of oesophageal varices.

Endoscopic: Upper GI endoscopy for definitive diagnosis ± management of upper GI bleeds. Adrenaline or sclerosant injection, clipping, photocoagulation or diathermy or a combination for bleeding ulcers. Varices are treated by band ligation or injection sclerotherapy.

Radiological: Embolisation of the bleeding site may be possible, e.g. in those unfit for surgery. Transjugular intrahepatic portocaval shunts can be performed in variceal haemorrhage uncontrolled by endoscopic means.

Gastrointestinal haemorrhage, upper (continued)

Surgical: For life-threatening bleeding, failure of endoscopic treatment (10–12%) or coexisting need for surgery, e.g. perforation. The procedure depends on site and cause, e.g. under-running of duodenal ulcer, in gastric ulcers partial gastrectomy may be required.

COMPLICATIONS

Anaemia, collapse and hypovolaemic shock.

PROGNOSIS

Depends on cause; if severe GI bleeds, aggressive resuscitation and early intervention improve outcome. The Rockall score (see table below) identifies patients at risk of adverse outcome. Higher mortality in older age groups (~14%) and those presenting with haemorrhagic shock (~30%), coagulopathy and cardiovascular disease. Recurrent bleeding can occur in upto 20% of patients after endoscopic therapy.

Rockall risk scoring system				
Variable	0	1	2	3
Age	<60 years	60–79 years	>80 years	
BP/Pulse	No shock	Pulse >100	SBP <100	
Comorbidity	None		CCF	Renal failure
			IHD	Liver failure
				Metastatic cancer
Diagnosis	Mallory–Weiss tear	All other causes	GI cancer	
Evidence of bleeding	None		Blood, adherent clot, spurting vessel	

Note: <3 carries good prognosis, >8 have a high risk of mortality.

Gastro-oesophageal reflux disease (GORD)

DEFINITION
Excessive reflux of gastric content into the oesophagus that causes symptoms and/or mucosal injury.

AETIOLOGY
Frequent and inappropriate transient lower oesophageal sphincter relaxations and disruption of mechanisms that prevent reflux (the physiological lower oesophageal sphincter, mucosal rosette, angle of His, diaphragmatic crura, intra-abdominal portion of oesophagus). Also contributing can be inefficient oesophageal antegrade peristalsis and impaired gastric motility/emptying.

ASSOCIATIONS/RISK FACTORS
Hiatus hernia, obesity, pregnancy, caffeine, fat or alcohol, smoking ($\downarrow$ lower oesophageal sphincter pressure), drugs, e.g. tricyclic antidepressants, $\uparrow$ gastric volume (large meal), systemic sclerosis.

EPIDEMIOLOGY
Common, 10–20% of adults in Western societies experience heartburn; of these approximately one-third will have evidence of GORD.

HISTORY
Typical: Retrosternal or epigastric discomfort or heartburn aggravated by lying supine, bending, alcohol or large meals, relieved by antacids, mass regurgitation of gastric contents or waterbrash.
Atypical: Chest pain, back pain, chronic wheeze or cough, especially at night, hoarse voice, halitosis.

EXAMINATION
Usually normal. Occasionally, epigastric tenderness, wheeze, dysphonia.

PATHOLOGY/PATHOGENESIS
Prolonged reflux of acid and bile causes oesophageal mucosal inflammation, erosions and ulceration. Chronic reflux may result in a fibrosis and stricture formation. Metaplasia of the lower oesophagus may occur with replacement of squamous epithelium by columnar, intestinal-type epithelium (Barrett's oesophagus) – a pre-malignant condition.

INVESTIGATIONS
Endoscopy: Often poor correlation between symptoms and endoscopic findings. Oesophagitis (seen in <50% with typical GORD symptoms); severity is graded by the modified Savary–Millar classification (1: erythema, 2: isolated erosions, 3: confluent erosions or superficial ulcers without stenosis, 4: deep ulceration, stricture formation) or the Los Angeles classification (grades A–D).
Barium swallow: Can show structural abnormalities (e.g. hiatus hernia, stricture).
Oesophageal manometry and 24-hour pH monitoring: Manometry assesses oesophageal peristalsis and enables placement of the pH probe above the LES. pH studies determine the temporal relationship between symptoms and oesophageal pH (significant reflux if pH <4 for >4.7% of time).

MANAGEMENT
Conservative: Lifestyle changes, weight loss, elevating head of bed, avoidance of provoking factors, stopping smoking, avoiding large meals late in the evening.
Medical: Antacids or alginates, H2 receptor antagonists and proton pump inhibitors.
Surgical: Antireflux surgery for those with symptoms/complications despite optimal medical management or in those intolerant of medication. Laparoscopic fundoplication, e.g. Nissen fundoplication: After a posterior hiatal repair, the fundus of the stomach is wrapped 360° around the lower oesophagus and held with seromuscular sutures. Modifications of this method include partial fundoplications, e.g. Toupet (270° wrap).
Endoscopic: Allows for stricture dilatation or surveillance of Barrett's oesophagus.

Gastro-oesophageal reflux disease (GORD) (continued)

COMPLICATIONS

Oesophageal ulceration, stricture, Barrett's oesophagus and oesophageal adenocarcinoma. Reflux asthma, cough and laryngitis syndromes. From surgery: dysphagia (3–8%, mostly temporary), gas bloat syndrome (difficulty belching), ↑ flatus, recurrent symptoms, rarely oesophageal perforation, pneumothorax, splenic injury.

PROGNOSIS

Fifty per cent respond to lifestyle measures alone. Drug therapy is effective, although withdrawal is often associated with relapse. Antireflux surgery offers effective symptom control in 85–90% of patients.

Hernia, hiatus

DEFINITION

Herniation of contents of the abdominal cavity, most commonly stomach, through the oesophageal hiatus of the diaphragm into the mediastinum (Fig. 29).

Type I (sliding): The gastro-oesophageal junction (GOJ) is above the diaphragm.

Type II (rolling/para-oesophageal): Defect in the phreno-oesophageal membrane and the GOJ does not move but the gastric fundus is the lead point of herniation.

Type III: Combination of Types I and II.

Type IV: Large defect with herniation of other organs such as colon, pancreas.

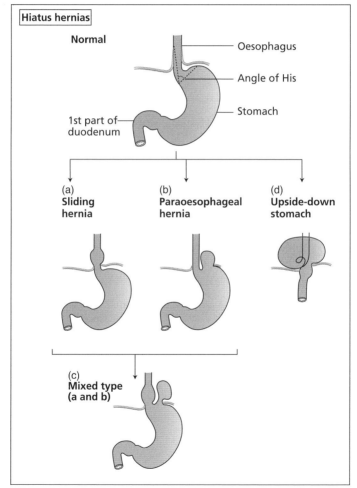

Figure 29 Types of hiatus herniae.

Hernia, hiatus (continued)

AETIOLOGY

Congenital or acquired, e.g. thinning and increased laxity of the phreno-oesophageal ligament with age. Associated with obesity, gastro-oesophageal reflux disease (GORD), chronic oesophagitis.

EPIDEMIOLOGY

Type I is the most common, ↑ frequency with age. Ninety-five per cent are sliding and 5% are rolling.

HISTORY

Many asymptomatic. Reflux symptoms of heartburn, indigestion, postprandial fullness and regurgitation.

EXAMINATION

In general, there are no signs of a hiatus hernia, unless complications develop.

INVESTIGATIONS

Endoscopy: Diagnosis of hernia and/or complications, e.g. oesophagitis, ulceration, Barrett's oesophagus.

Radiology: CXR (large hernias can appear as a gastric air bubble behind the heart), barium swallow or meal.

High-resolution manometry: Can diagnose sliding hernias.

MANAGEMENT

Modification of lifestyle factors: E.g. weight loss, avoiding late meals.

Medical: Antacids, H2 antagonists, proton pump inhibitors.

Surgical: Necessary only in the minority of patients. Indications include complications of reflux disease despite aggressive treatment, those with mass reflux or pulmonary complications and para-oesophageal hernia that are more at risk of incarceration and strangulation. Now commonly repaired laparoscopically. Surgery involves hernia reduction, crural repair with or without prosthetic reinforcement, combined with antireflux fundoplication, e.g. Nissen's. Mesh repairs are controversial, as there is risk of infection, stricture and mesh erosion.

COMPLICATIONS

Oesophageal complications: Oesophagitis, erosions or ulceration, strictures, Barrett's oesophagus.

Other: Rarely, incarceration of para-oesophageal hernia, strangulation or perforation. Para-oesophageal hernia can enlarge with time, and sometimes progress to where the entire stomach lies within the thoracic cavity (upside-down stomach); there are respiratory problems.

Of surgery: High recurrence rates in large hiatus hernias (5–30%). Of mesh repairs: infection, stricturing, visceral erosion.

PROGNOSIS

Generally good, with most not causing severe problems. Sliding hernias have a better prognosis than rolling hernias.

Oesophageal carcinoma

DEFINITION

Malignant tumour arising in the oesophageal mucosa. Two major histological types: squamous cell carcinoma and adenocarcinoma.

AETIOLOGY

Squamous: Alcohol, tobacco, certain nutritional deficiencies (vitamins, trace elements), HPV infection, achalasia, Paterson–Kelly (Plummer–Vinson) syndrome, tylosis (Howel–Evans syndrome), scleroderma, coeliac disease, lye stricture, history of previous thoracic radiotherapy or upper aerodigestive squamous cancer, dietary nitrosamines.

Adenocarcinoma: GORD, Barrett's oesophagus (intestinal metaplasia of the distal oesophageal mucosa with ~0.5–0.7% incidence of adenocarcinoma per year).

EPIDEMIOLOGY

Eighth most common malignancy (7000–8000 per year in the UK). 3–4:1 male:female. Worldwide, squamous carcinoma is more common, with considerable geographic variation (high incidence in northern China, Iran and southern Russia). Adenocarcinoma is more common in westernised countries (65% cases in the UK), increasing by 5–10% per year. Peak incidence 60–70 years.

HISTORY

Early: Asymptomatic/symptoms of reflux. Later: dysphagia, initially worse for solids, regurgitation, cough or choking after food, pain (odynophagia), weight loss, fatigue, voice hoarseness (may indicate recurrent laryngeal nerve palsy).

EXAMINATION

No physical signs may be evident; signs of weight loss. With metastatic disease there may be supraclavicular lymphadenopathy and hepatomegaly. Respiratory signs may be due to aspiration or direct tracheobronchial involvement.

PATHOLOGY/PATHOGENESIS

Squamous cell carcinomas are more common in the mid-upper oesophagus. Adenocarcinomas usually develop in the lower oesophagus or, increasingly, in the gastro-oesophageal junction (GOJ). Barrett's intestinal metaplasia can progress to low-grade dysplasia, high-grade dysplasia and invasive carcinoma. Spread is typically initially direct (oesophagus has no serosa) and longitudinal via an extensive network of submucosal lymphatics to tracheobronchial, mediastinal, coeliac, gastric or cervical nodes. Rare oesophageal tumours include lymphoma, melanoma and leiomyosarcoma.

INVESTIGATIONS

Endoscopy: Tumour location and biopsy. Early high-grade dysplasia and cancer detection is improved by endoscopic techniques such as narrow band imaging or magnification and chromoendoscopy. Endoscopic ultrasound for T (depth of tumour involvement) and N (perioesophageal node) involvement.

Imaging: Barium swallow, CT (chest, abdomen, pelvis) and PET can detect previously occult distant metastases.

Other: Bronchoscopy (if risk of tracheo-bronchial invasion), bone scan if symptoms of bony involvement. Laparoscopy and peritoneal washings, thoracoscopy. Careful cardiac and respiratory assessment if surgery is planned.

MANAGEMENT

Best managed at specialist centres with multidisciplinary expertise. For early (mucosal) localised disease, endoscopic therapies are increasing, e.g. endoscopic mucosal resection, endoscopic submucosal dissection. Surgical: Only ~30% are suitable for surgical resection. Neoadjuvant chemoradiotherapy (e.g. cisplatin, 5-fluorouracil) can be beneficial in downstaging tumours prior to surgery.

Oesophageal carcinoma (continued)

Surgery: Operative approach depends on tumour location and extent of proposed lymphadenectomy.

■ *Transthoracic approach*: Ivor–Lewis right thoracotomy and laparotomy (mid-lower third tumours).
■ *Transhiatal approach*: Laparotomy, blunt dissection of the thoracic oesophagus and cervical incision for oesophagogastric anastomosis (upper third tumours).
■ *McKeown tri-incisional (abdomen, right chest and neck) approach*.
  Reconstruction is by formation of a conduit, most commonly gastric, based on a vascular pedicle of the right gastroepiploic and right gastric arteries, less commonly colon or jejunum (for GOJ tumours with significant gastric involvement). A pyloroplasty for gastric drainage and feeding jejunostomy for postoperative enteral nutrition are often performed. Some studies have shown improved survival with more extensive (three-field as opposed to two-field) lymphadenectomy.
■ *Minimally invasive approaches*: Increasingly used, i.e. laparoscopic and thoracoscopic dissection.

Radiotherapy/Chemotherapy: Squamous cell carcinomas are more radiosensitive than adenocarcinomas. Radical radio- or chemoradiotherapy can be performed in localised disease if patients are unfit for surgery. Neoadjuvant and adjuvant chemotherapy using a cisplatin-based regimen is used where tolerated.

Palliation: It is tailored to individual patient's tumour and symptoms. Luminal recannulisation can be achieved by expandable stents or laser ablation or photodynamic therapy techniques. Radiotherapy and/or chemotherapy is associated with variable response rates, e.g. epirubicin, cisplatin and 5-fluorouracil.

COMPLICATIONS

Of tumour: Malnutrition, aspiration pneumonia, haematemesis, oesophago-bronchial fistula; of metastatic disease: ascites, pleural effusions.

Of oesophagectomy: Mortality <5% in specialised centres; morbidity up to 40%. Pulmonary complications are the most common, e.g. atelectasis, pneumonia. Serious complications include anastomotic leakage (5–15%) or conduit failure; others: chylothorax, recurrent laryngeal nerve damage.

PROGNOSIS

Depends on stage. Overall 5-year survival is 20–25%; for advanced disease, 5-year survival <5%.

Oesophageal perforation

DEFINITION

Rupture of the oesphogeal wall, often associated with spillage of contents into the mediastinum.

AETIOLOGY

Spontaneous: Boerhaave's syndrome. Barogenic disruption of the oesophageal wall in the absence of preexisting pathology, most commonly caused by forceful vomiting, occasionally severe Valsalva manoeuvres, e.g. parturition, heavy weightlifting etc.

Iatrogenic: During upper GI endoscopy, (e.g. during dilatation).

Trauma: Penetrating or rarely blunt injury, foreign bodies.

Caustic: Acid or alkali 'lye' ingestion cause liquefactive or coagulative necrosis and risk of perforation.

EPIDEMIOLOGY

Rare, Boerhaave's syndrome: males > females (4 : 1).

HISTORY

Sudden severe chest pain following an episode of raised intra-abdominal pressure; most commonly vomiting. A high index of suspicion is required.

EXAMINATION

Tachycardia, tachypnoea, subcutaneous emphysema (Mackler's triad: subcutaneous emphysema, vomiting and chest pain), epigastric tenderness. Haematemesis is uncommon.

PATHOLOGY/PATHOGENESIS

Spontaneous perforations tend to occur in the distal oesophagus posterolaterally as a longitudinal tear. Negative intrathoracic pressure draws gastric contents into the mediastinum/pleural cavity causing a chemical mediastinitis followed rapidly by severe sepsis.

Ten to twenty per cent are associated with underlying oesophageal abnormalities, e.g. peptic ulceration, malignancy or infection.

INVESTIGATIONS

Imaging: CXR and CT scan can show pleural effusion, air-fluid collections, pneumomediastinum, pneumothorax or subcutaneous emphysema. Water-soluble contrast swallow to detect leak (false negative ~10%).

Oesophagogastroscopy: Should only be performed by experienced endoscopists in an appropriate centre. Can confirm the site, extent of injury and any underlying pathology. Also enables placement of nasogastric tube for gastric drainage.

MANAGEMENT

Emergency: Resuscitation (ABC) – oxygen, respiratory and cardiovascular support, intravenous fluids, urinary catheterisation, strict fluid balance, intravenous proton-pump inhibitors, early intensivist review, multidisciplinary care and close monitoring in an HDU/ITU setting.

Control of sepsis: Nil by mouth, commencement of broad-spectrum antibiotics and antifungal agents, adequate chest drainage and maintenance of nutrition. Ideally managed in a specialist oesophagogastric unit.

Non-operative management: Only in selected cases with early recognition, limited injury and minimal contamination or cervical perforations. Endoscopic clipping of some early perforations is reported.

Surgery: Thoracotomy, drainage and debridement of contaminated area and devitalised oesophageal tissue. Treatment options include:
- primary repair ± reinforcement, e.g. with flap of pleura or intercostal muscle (can be prone to failure and leak);
- repair over T-tube – allows formation of controlled oesophagocutaneous fistula;

Oesophageal perforation (continued)

- oesophageal resection with immediate or delayed reconstruction (major undertaking);
- exclusion and diversion – formation of oesophagostomy; needs later reconstruction. Formation of feeding jejunostomy for enteral feeding should be performed.

COMPLICATIONS
Mediastinitis, subcutaneous emphysema, pleural effusion, severe sepsis, shock, multiorgan failure and death.

PROGNOSIS
High mortality, overall ~20% (10% with early diagnosis and treatment; up to 60% in late presentations).

Peptic ulcer disease

DEFINITION
Ulceration of areas of the GI tract caused by exposure to gastric acid and pepsin. Most commonly gastric and duodenal (can also occur in oesophagus and Meckel's diverticulum).

AETIOLOGY
Cause is an imbalance between damaging action of acid and pepsin and mucosal protective mechanisms. There is a strong correlation with *Helicobacter pylori* infection, but it is unclear how the organism causes formation of ulcers.
Common: Very strong association with *H. pylori* (present in 95% of duodenal and 70–80% of gastric ulcers), NSAID use.
Rare: Zollinger–Ellison syndrome (ZE).

EPIDEMIOLOGY
Common. Annual incidence is about 1–4/1000. More common in males. Duodenal ulcers have a mean age in the thirties, while gastric ulcers have a mean age in the fifties. *H. pylori* is usually acquired in childhood and the prevalence is roughly equivalent to age in years.

HISTORY
Epigastric abdominal pain: Relieved by antacids.
Symptoms have a variable relationship to food:
- if worse soon after eating, more likely to be gastric ulcers and
- if worse several hours later, more likely to be duodenal.
May present with complications (e.g. haematemesis, melaena).

EXAMINATION
May be no physical findings.
Epigastric tenderness.
Signs of complications (e.g. anaemia, succession splash in pyloric stenosis).

INVESTIGATIONS
Bloods: FBC (for anaemia), amylase (to exclude pancreatitis), U&Es, clotting screen (if GI bleeding); LFT, cross-match if actively bleeding. Secretin test, if ZE is suspected: i.v. secretin causes a rise in serum gastrin in ZE patients but not controls.
Endoscopy: Four quadrant gastric ulcer biopsies to rule out malignancy; duodenal ulcers need not be biopsied.
Rockall scoring (see *Gastrointestinal Haemorrhage, Upper*): Severity scoring after a GI bleed: <3, carry good prognosis; >8, have a high risk of mortality.
Testing for *H. pylori*:
- ^{13}C-Urea breath test: Radio-labelled urea given by mouth and ^{13}C detected in the expired air.
- Serology: IgG antibody against *H. pylori*; confirms exposure but not eradication.
- Stool antigen test. *Campylobacter*-like organism test.
- Gastric biopsy is placed with a substrate of urea and a pH indicator, if *H. pylori* is present, ammonia is produced from the urea and there is a colour change (yellow to red).
Histology of biopsies: Difficult to visualise *H. pylori*, so of limited value.
Imaging: Erect CXR or CT to investigate for evidence of perforation.

MANAGEMENT
Acute: Resuscitation if perforated or bleeding, and proceeding endoscopic or surgical treatment.
Endoscopy: Haemostasis by injection sclerotherapy, laser or electrocoagulation.
Surgical: If perforated, ulcer can be oversewn or an omental patch can be placed over it. Haemorrhage is controlled by suturing the affected vessels (often the gastroduodenal artery). In chronic cases where ulcer-related bleeding cannot be controlled, partial gastrectomy and/or vagotomy and sometimes trans-arterial embolisation can be performed.

Peptic ulcer disease (continued)

Medical: *H. pylori* eradication with 'triple therapy' for 1–2 weeks: Various combinations are recommended made up of one of PPI/ranitidine bismuth sulphate and two antibiotics (e.g. clarithromycin + amoxicillin; metronidazole + tetracycline).

If not associated with *H. pylori*: Treat with PPIs or H2-antagonists. Stop NSAID use (especially diclofenac); use misoprostol (prostaglandin E1 analogue), if NSAID use is necessary.

COMPLICATIONS

Rate of major complication is 1% per year including haemorrhage (haematemesis, melaena, iron deficiency anaemia), perforation, obstruction/pyloric stenosis (due to scarring), pancreatitis.

PROGNOSIS

Overall lifetime risk ~10%. Generally good as peptic ulcers associated with *H. pylori* can be cured by eradication.

Pyloric stenosis

DEFINITION

Hypertrophy of the pylorus in infants, resulting in gastric outflow obstruction.

AETIOLOGY

Poorly understood, may be related to abnormalities in pyloric innervation, smooth muscle cells or interstitial cells of Cajal that result in hypertrophy and hyperplasia of the pyloric smooth muscle.

Associated with jaundice in 2% due to defective hepatic glucuronyl transferase activity, which resolves after surgery.

EPIDEMIOLOGY

Annual incidence $\sim$3 per 1000; less common in African/Asian. Male: female ratio is 4 : 1; typically presents in the first 2–12 weeks of life but can occur later in premature babies.

HISTORY

Baby develops forceful 'projectile' vomiting of milk; not bilious, but if prolonged, may be blood stained due to associated oesophagitis. Although initially well and appearing hungry, the baby with time becomes lethargic and dehydrated.

EXAMINATION

Baby may appear well, or underweight, and show signs of dehydration (5–15% body weight, sunken fontanelles, dry mucous membranes, poor skin turgor). Abdominal examination can show gastric peristaltic waves from the left to right upper quadrant. The hypertrophied pylorus may be felt as a pyloric 'tumour', an olive-sized firm lump in the epigastrium.

INVESTIGATIONS

Bloods: U&Es, capillary gases to determine metabolic derangement (metabolic alkalosis with $\downarrow K^+$ and $\downarrow Cl^-$, the latter giving an indication of the severity of dehydration.

Imaging: Ultrasound demonstrates the thickened pylorus muscle and narrowed pyloric canal (wall thickness > 4 mm; total diameter > 10 mm; length > 18 mm).

MANAGEMENT

General: Correction of biochemical abnormalities and rehydration is carried out with iv fluids prior to any surgery (if not, there is a risk of apnoea post anaesthesia because of loss of respiratory drive from both $\downarrow H^+$ due to alkalosis and $\downarrow CO_2$ due to ventilation). An NG tube is inserted to prevent aspiration of gastric contents.

Surgical: Ramstedt's pyloromyotomy is the definitive procedure undertaken usually in a specialist paediatric surgical department. Can be performed by open epigastric or circumumbilical incisions or laparoscopically. The pylorus is identified, the serosa cut by knife or diathermy and the circular muscle then split along the anterior wall down to the mucosa. The stomach is then filled with air to ensure that the mucosa has not been perforated (if this is the case, the defect should be sutured and an omental patch placed over the mucosa).

COMPLICATIONS

Malnutrition, dehydration, hypochloraemic hypokalaemic metabolic alkalosis, gastritis and oesophagitis, aspiration and respiratory distress syndrome.

Of surgery: mucosal perforation, wound infection, incisional hernia. Post surgery, persistent vomiting is seen in $\sim$10% but usually settles (may be due to reflux disease).

PROGNOSIS

Usually excellent. Morbidity <3% and mortality <0.5% in those undergoing surgery.

Volvulus, gastric

DEFINITION

Gastric volvulus is abnormal rotation of all or part of the stomach >180°, resulting in obstruction. Classified as subdiaphragmatic ($^1/_3$) or supradiaphragmatic ($^2/_3$, associated with diaphragmatic defects), or on the basis of axis of rotation:

- *Organoaxial*: Around a longitudinal axis through the gastroesophageal junction and the pylorus,
- *Mesenteroaxial*: Rotation along an axis perpendicular to its longitudinal axis.
- Combination types can occur.

AETIOLOGY

Subdiaphragmatic: Abnormal laxity of the gastrosplenic, gastroduodenal, gastrohepatic and gastrophrenic ligaments (more common in adults).

Supradiaphragmatic: Congenital or acquired anatomical abnormalities in the diaphragm, paraoesophageal hernia.

ASSOCIATIONS/RISK FACTORS

Please see **Aetiology**.

EPIDEMIOLOGY

Organoaxial is the most common type; combined cases are rare. Ten to twenty per cent cases occur in children, usually <1 year. Rare in adults <50 years.

HISTORY

Acute volvulus presents as an emergency with severe epigastric or chest pain and non-productive retching; occasionally haematemesis or respiratory distress. Chronic volvulus: epigastric pain and fullness after meals; in children, feeding problems and growth failure.

EXAMINATION

Upper abdominal distention and tenderness.
Borchardt's triad is pain, retching and inability to pass a nasogastric tube.

INVESTIGATIONS

CXR: Gas bubble behind the heart if intrathoracic.
AXR: Gas shadow of very distended viscus.
Barium swallow or CT scan: Diagnosis of acute cases.

MANAGEMENT

General: Resuscitation and a trial of nasogastric decompression. Endoscopic reduction is controversial but can be attempted as a temporising measure in patients who are high risk for surgery.

Surgical: Open or laparoscopic reduction of the volvulus. An assessment is made of viability of the stomach, and partial, subtotal or total gastrectomy may be required if gangrenous. To prevent recurrence, anterior gastropexy is performed with repair of any associated diaphragmatic defect.

COMPLICATIONS

Vascular compromise with strangulation and necrosis, ulceration, haemorrhage and perforation.

PROGNOSIS

Non-operative mortality rate, especially in acute presentations, is high, usually due to delayed diagnosis. With appropriate management now mortality <16%.

Benign prostatic hyperplasia

DEFINITION
Slowly progressive nodular hyperplasia of the periurethral (transitional) zone of the prostate gland, the most frequent cause of lower urinary tract symptoms in adult males.

AETIOLOGY
Precise cause unknown; related to age, testosterone and dihydrotestosterone exposure. Epithelial and stromal hyperplasia of the periurethral transition zone of the prostate, becomes surrounded by a false capsule of compressed peripheral zone glandular tissue.

EPIDEMIOLOGY
Common; 70% of men aged 70 years have histological benign prostate hypherplasia (BPH), with 50% of these experiencing significant symptoms, West > Far East, Afro-Carribean > Caucasian.

HISTORY
Obstructive symptoms: Hesitancy, poor or intermittent stream, terminal dribbling and incomplete emptying.
Irritative/storage symptoms: Frequency, urgency, urge incontinence and nocturia. The International Prostate Symptom Score is a questionnaire to assess symptoms and response to treatment.
Acute retention: Sudden inability to pass urine, associated with severe pain.
Chronic retention: Painless, frequency with passage of small volumes of urine, especially at night.

EXAMINATION
On digital rectal examination, the prostate is often enlarged; however, there is often poor correlation between the size and symptoms, and if nodular, prostate carcinoma should be suspected.
Acute retention: Suprapubic pain and a distended palpable bladder.
Chronic retention: A large distended painless bladder (residual volumes > 1 L), and there may be signs of renal failure.

INVESTIGATIONS
Bloods: U&Es for renal function, PSA.
Urine: For microscopy, culture and sensitivity.
Imaging: Ultrasound imaging of the renal tract to check for dilatation of the upper urinary tract. Bladder scanning to measure pre- and postvoiding volumes.
Transrectal ultrasound: To measure prostate size and guide biopsies.
Histology: Epithelial and stromal hyperplasia of the periurethal transition zone of the prostate, becomes surrounded by a false capsule of compressed peripheral zone glandular tissue.
Flexible cystoscopy: To visualise the bladder outlet and bladder changes (e.g. trabeculation).
Others: Urinary flow studies (flowmetry).

MANAGEMENT
Depends on the severity of symptoms and the presence of complications.
Emergency: In acute retention, urinary catheterisation.
Conservative: If mild, 'watchful waiting' may be appropriate with symptom monitoring using the IPSS questionnaire.
Medical: Selective α-blockers relax smooth muscle of the internal (bladder neck) sphincter and the prostate capsule (e.g. alfuzosin, tamsulosin). 5 α-reductase inhibitors act by inhibiting conversion of testosterone to dihydrotestosterone (e.g. finasteride); reduce prostate size by ~20%, but may take time to show improvement.
Surgery: Transurethral resection of the prostate (TURP) involves resection from within the prostatic urethra; may be achieved using a variety of methods, e.g. electrocautery, laser. Open prostatectomy (retropubic or suprapubic approaches) is usually reserved for very large glands (>60 g); may be performed by open surgery, laparoscopy or robot-assisted surgery.

Benign prostatic hyperplasia (continued)

COMPLICATIONS

Recurrent urinary infections, acute or chronic urinary retention, urinary stasis and bladder diverticulae or stone development, obstructive renal failure, post-obstructive diuresis.

From TURP: Retrograde ejaculation (common), haemorrhage (primary, reactionary or secondary 2–10%), clot retention, more rarely incontinence, TUR syndrome (seizures or cardiovascular collapse caused by hypervolaemia and hyponatraemia due to absorption of glycine irrigation fluid), urinary infection, erectile dysfunction; late: urethral stricture.

PROGNOSIS

Mild symptoms may be improved by medical therapies, but those with marked symptoms usually obtain significant relief from surgical intervention.

Bladder cancer

DEFINITION
Malignancy of bladder urothelium.
Majority are transitional cell carcinoma, with a 'field change' of the bladder epithelium. Others include squamous cell carcinomas associated with chronic inflammation (e.g. in schistosomiasis), or adenocarcinomas arising in the urachal remnant. Rarer are small cell carcinomas (neuroendocrine), leiomyosarcomas and carcinosarcomas.

AETIOLOGY
Several genetic abnormalities are associated, including chromosome 9 mutations in $p15$, $p16$ in superficial tumours. Others include mutations in $p53$, $p21$, ras, c-myc and c-jun.

ASSOCIATIONS/RISK FACTORS
Tobacco, exposure to naphthylamines and benzidine in dye, rubber and leather industries, cyclophosphamide treatment (10% risk after 12 years of exposure), pelvic irradiation (e.g. for cervical carcinoma), chronic UTIs, schistosomiasis; early menopause has been shown to increase risk by 50%. Patent urachus is associated with adenocarcinoma.

EPIDEMIOLOGY
~2% of cancers, second most common cancer of the genitourinary system, men 2–3 times more commonly affected than women, rare <50 years, mean age at diagnosis in sixties.

HISTORY
Most commonly, painless macroscopic haematuria. Other symptoms include urinary frequency, urgency or nocturia, recurrent UTIs. Rarely, pain due to clot retention, ureteral obstruction or extension to pelvis.

EXAMINATION
Often no signs.
If advanced, mass or lymphadenopathy may be palpable.

INVESTIGATIONS
Urine: Cytology microscopy and culture.
Cystoscopy: Allows visualisation of the tumour and biopsy or removal.
USS, IVU: To assess upper and lower urinary tract, as tumours can be multifocal (Fig. 30).
CT or MRI scan: For staging.
TNM staging: *Tis*, flat carcinoma-*in-situ*; T1a, papillary tumour above lamina propria; T1, submucosal invasion of lamina propria; T2, invasion of muscle; T3, invasion of perivesical tissue; T4, invasion of adjacent organs or pelvic wall; N, nodal involvement; M, metastases. 70% are superficial at the time of diagnosis.
Three grades: G1, well differentiated; G2, moderately differentiated and G3, poorly differentiated.

MANAGEMENT
Depends on stage and grade of tumour.
Superficial tumours (Tis, T1): Transurethral resection of bladder tumour (TURBT). Intravesical chemotherapy with mitomycin C or intravesical immunotherapy with BCG instillation to reduce recurrence rates. Close follow-up with repeat cystoscopy and bladder cytology every 3 months for 2 years, then every 6 months for 2 years, then yearly. High-grade T1 tumours may be best treated by cystectomy. Upper tract disease may require nephro-ureterectomy.
Invasive tumours (T2 and above): Radical cystectomy if localised (includes hysterectomy and bilateral salpingo-oopherectomy in women, cystoprostatectomy in men with urinary diversion by an ileal conduit or orthoptic reconstruction and pelvic lymph node dissection). Specialised centres can perform laparoscopic or robotic-assisted procedures.

Bladder cancer (continued)

Radiotherapy or chemotherapy: Radical radiotherapy is an alternative if unfit for surgery, with salvage cystectomy for relapse post radiotherapy. Palliative radiotherapy ± chemotherapy is used in metastatic disease, e.g. M-VAC (methotrexate, vinblastine, doxorubicin and cisplatin).

COMPLICATIONS
Haematuria and clot retention, hydronephrosis due to ureteric orifice obstruction.
Surgery: *Early:* Ileus, infection, haemorrhage, bowel obstruction, rectal injury.
Late: Bowel obstruction, pyelonephritis, nephrolithiasis, hernia, fistula.
Radiotherapy: Postradiotherapy cystitis, haemorrhage, bladder contraction.

PROGNOSIS
Following TURBT, 75% will develop other tumours, but only 10% progress to invasive disease. Five-year survival for T1 90–100%, T2 ~70%, T3 30–65%, T4 10–20%. With distant metastases ~6% 5-year survival.

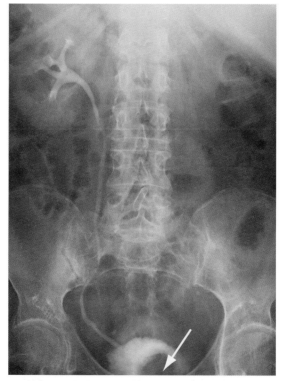

Figure 30 Intravenous urogram (IVU) showing a filling defect (bladder cancer) and right standing column.

Epididymitis and orchitis

DEFINITION
Inflammation of the epididymis or testes (orchitis). Sixty per cent of epididymitis is associated with orchitis and most cases of orchitis with epididymitis.

AETIOLOGY
Majority of cases are infective in origin, although one-third are idiopathic.
Bacterial: <35 years, most commonly *Chlamydia* or *gonococcus*. For >35 years, most common organisms are coliforms. Rarely: tuberculosis, tertiary syphilis.
Viral: Mumps (orchitis often follows recent parotitis), coxsackie, EBV.
Fungal: E.g. *Candida* if immunocompromised.
Inflammatory disorders: Behcet's disease, post-vasectomy.
May be associated with underlying testicular tumour.

EPIDEMIOLOGY
Common. Obviously only affects males. ~50% are 20–30 years.

HISTORY
Painful, swollen and tender testes or epididymis (usually unilateral).
Onset is less acute than testicular torsion – the most important differential.
Penile discharge may occur (especially in bacterial forms), fever.
Important to enquire about sexual history and any history of parotitis.

EXAMINATION
Erythematous and oedematous scrotum.
Swollen and tender epididymis and/or testis.
Walking or even eliciting a cremaster reflex may be painful.
Palpate the parotid glands for parotid enlargement or tenderness.
Pyrexia.
Prehn's sign: Elevation of scrotum alleviates pain in epididymitis and orchitis but not testicular torsion.

INVESTIGATIONS
Mid-stream urine: MC&S, early morning urine collection (for AFB if risk of TB).
Blood: ↑WCC, ↑CRP, U&E, mumps serology.
Testicular Doppler ultrasound: To exclude torsion, local abscess.
Abdominal ultrasound: May be necessary to exclude bladder outflow obstruction.
Following treatment of acute episode: Repeat imaging after resolution should be performed to exclude testicular malignancy.

MANAGEMENT
Medical: *Antibiotics if appropriate.
Young patients: Quinolones with activity against chlamydia (ofloxacin, levofloxacin) for 2 weeks. Alternatively, consider doxycycline. Analgesia and scrotal support.
Older patients: Quinolones (e.g. ciprofloxacin) for 2 weeks.
If TB is suspected, antituberculous regimen is necessary.
Analgesia and scrotal support.
Follow-up is recommended to exclude testicular malignancy.
Surgical: Exploration of scrotum may be necessary if testicular torsion cannot be excluded or if an abscess or pyocoele develops that requires drainage. May be necessary in cases of tuberculous cases not responding to medical treatment.
Public health: Contact tracing especially if individual is sexually active.

---

* There is no evidence to support the use of steroids to prevent permanent occlusion of epididymal ducts and infertility.

Epididymitis and orchitis (continued)

COMPLICATIONS

Pain, abscess; if untreated, risk of spreading infection and Fournier's gangrene. Minimal risk to fertility if unilateral and treated. Testicular atrophy occurs in 50% of mumps orchitis (if bilateral disease, increased risk of sterility).

PROGNOSIS

Generally good if treated. May take up to 2 months for swelling to completely resolve.

Hydrocoele

DEFINITION

A fluid collection between the parietal and visceral layers of the tunica vaginalis in the scrotum. A hydrocoele of the cord (rare) is a fluid collection in part of the processus closed off to the peritoneal cavity and tunica vaginalis.

AETIOLOGY

Congenital (or communicating, due to a patent processus vaginalis, the peritoneum that follows the descent of the testicle into the scrotum, with failure of obliteration leaving a small communication and peritoneal fluid tracts into the tunica vaginalis) or acquired: most commonly idiopathic.

Secondary causes: Infection, e.g. epididymo-orchitis or parasitic infection with *Wuchereria bancrofti* or filariasis, tumour, trauma or underlying torsion of testicle or testicular appendage.

ASSOCIATIONS/RISK FACTORS

Indirect inguinal hernias in children. Epididymo-orchitis is a common cause in the UK. Filariasis is the cause of large hydrocoeles in countries of high prevalence.

EPIDEMIOLOGY

A patent processus vaginalis is very common in male infants, obliterating in most children by the age of two. Hydrocoeles are common in older men. *Filariasis* is the most common cause in adults worldwide.

HISTORY

Scrotal swelling. Usually asymptomatic, but may be associated with pain or urinary symptoms due to underlying cause.

EXAMINATION

Scrotal swelling (firm or doughy), in which it is possible to get above the swelling; usually trans-illuminates and it is difficult to feel the associated testicle as separate.

INVESTIGATIONS

Ultrasound: Shows anechoic fluid collection surrounding anterolateral aspect of the testis. Also used to examine testis for underlying tumours.

Urine: Dipstick, MSU for infection.

Blood: Markers of testicular tumours if suspected (αFP, β-HCG).

MANAGEMENT

In infants, most are resorbed spontaneously and ligation of the patent processus at the deep ring by an inguinal approach is only conducted after 1 year of age, often in association with repair of inguinal hernia. In adults, aspiration of the hydrocoele is not recommended, as it tends to re-accumulate, and may introduce infection or cause a haematocoele.

Surgical: In adults, a scrotal approach is usually used. Redundant tunica vaginalis can be excised and the remaining treated by a Jaboulay procedure whereby the sac is everted or Lord's procedure in which the sac is plicated.

Secondary hydrocoeles require treatment of the underlying cause.

COMPLICATIONS

Discomfort, scrotal swelling.

Of surgery: Infection, haematoma, injury to spermatic cord structures or nerves, recurrence.

PROGNOSIS

Idiopathic hydrocoeles tend to be chronic with recurrence rates 1%–2% following surgical treatment. Acute secondary hydrocoeles generally resolve once the predisposing factor has been treated.

Penile carcinoma

DEFINITION
Penile malignancy, most commonly squamous cell carcinoma of the penile skin.

AETIOLOGY
Chronic irritation is the main risk factor.
- Condyloma acuminata (human papilloma virus)
- Chronic infection of the foreskin (balanitis), smoking
- Balanitis xerotica obliterans (a form of lichen sclerosus, a chronic inflammatory condition of the glans or foreskin)
- Erythroplasia of Queyrat (a form of carcinoma *in situ* of the glans skin)
- Bowen's disease (intraepithelial carcinoma of the penile shaft).

EPIDEMIOLOGY
Rare in developed countries (<0.5% of adult male cancers). More common in Africa/South America. Most commonly seen in elderly men (50–70 years).

HISTORY
The patient may report a slowly enlarging lesion, often painless leading to a delay in seeking medical attention. There may be associated bleeding or discharge.

EXAMINATION
Most often occurs on the glans penis or inner surface of the foreskin, early as a painless red lesion, later as an exophytic or nodular growth or ulcer, often with secondary infection causing a discharge or offensive smell. Inguinal lymphadenopathy is present in up to 50%, often due to the associated infection or inflammation, with only 30–60% of these having evidence of tumour spread.

PATHOLOGY/PATHOGENESIS
These are squamous cell carcinomas, with three histological grades G1–G3. Jackson classification of Stage I: Localised to the glans or foreskin. Stage II: Involvement of the corpora. Stage III: Spread to inguinal nodes. Stage IV: Distant metastases. Also TNM staging. A variant is giant condyloma of Buschke–Löwenstein that spreads locally with a characteristic sharply defined deep margin.

INVESTIGATIONS
Biopsy: Punch or excisional biopsy to establish diagnosis (differential: condylomata acuminata, syphilitic chancre or rarely chancroid).
Imaging: CT or MRI scanning for evidence of spread. Sentinal lymph node biopsy.

MANAGEMENT
Localised disease: On the glans or Bowens disease on the shaft (carcinoma *in situ*) 5-fluorouracil cream, laser photocoagulation or cryosurgery.
Surgical: For early stage: wide local excision, Mohs microsurgery, stage I and II, partial penectomy with 2 cm proximal disease-free margins. In more advanced cases, total penectomy with formation of a perineal urethrostomy. Inguinal nodes: If impalpable, occult metastases in 20–25%. Palpable nodes may not be due to metastases. Bilateral lymphadenectomy if suspicious on scanning. More recently, sentinel node biopsy or limited inguinal node dissection superficial to the fascia lata.
Radiotherapy: Local for early-stage disease if the tumour is not large, invasive or involving the urethra, or as part of combined modality therapy for palliation of advanced-stage disease.
Chemotherapy: Usually restricted to cases of systemic spread; agents such as cisplatin and irinotecan used.
Prevention: Circumcision as a newborn reduces risk (number needed to treat to prevent one cancer in 909). Good hygiene and appropriate treatment of erythroplasia of Queyrat.

COMPLICATIONS

From surgery: Infection, lymphoedema, wound breakdown, urethral stricture. Psychological morbidity of penectomy.

PROGNOSIS

Often present late due to embarrassment/neglect. Five-year survival rate is >90% for *in situ* disease, 80% for invasive that has not spread to lymph nodes, approximately 50% with nodal involvement and <20% if distant metastases.

Prostate carcinoma

DEFINITION
Primary malignant neoplasm of the prostate gland. Majority are adenocarcinomas (95%) with a variable degree of differentiation.

AETIOLOGY
Unknown. See **Associations/Risk Factors**.

ASSOCIATIONS/RISK FACTORS
Age is the biggest risk factor. Race: Afro-Caribbean > Caucasian, and the former tend to present with more aggressive disease at a younger age. Geographic distribution: higher in North America and Europe, and low in the Far East. Family history: A gene on chromosome 1 implicated. Dietary factors: High fat, meat and alcohol consumption associated, ↓ with soy.

EPIDEMIOLOGY
Second most common cause of male cancer deaths. Annual incidence 50–70 per 100,000. Microfoci of cancer are found in 80% of men over 80 years on autopsy.

HISTORY
Often asymptomatic and detected on PSA testing.
Lower urinary tract obstruction: Frequency, hesitancy, poor stream, nocturia and terminal dribble.
Metastatic spread: Bone pain or spinal cord compression from bone metastases.
General symptoms of malignancy include malaise, anorexia and weight loss.

EXAMINATION
Digital rectal examination: Asymmetrical hard nodular prostate gland with loss of the midline sulcus.

INVESTIGATIONS
Blood: FBC, U&E, PSA, LFT and bone profile.
Prostate-specific antigen: Values are age-related and non-specific (maybe ↑ in benign prostatic hyperplasia, prostatitis, following catheterisation).
Trans-rectal ultrasound (TRUS) and needle biopsy: Digital rectal examination and PSA level guides decision whether to proceed with TRUS and biopsy. Various decision-making algorithms are used, for example:
  • patients with a PSA >10 ng/ml, regardless of digital rectal examination.
  • patients with a PSA 4–10 ng/ml and free PSA <30%.
  • patients with a palpable nodule on digital rectal examination.
Gleason score: Grading based on histology from biopsy; two scores are given based on predominant appearance, with maximum score of 5 + 5 (10).
CT/MRI scan: Assesses extent of local invasion and lymph node involvement.
Isotope bone scan: For bone metastases.
TNM staging system:
T1a: incidental <5% on TURP;
T1b: incidental >5% on TURP;
T1c: identified on needle biopsy;
T2: confined to prostate (a: one lobe; b: both lobes);
T3: extending through capsule;
T4: fixed tumour invading adjacent structures other than seminal vesicles;
N1: regional lymph nodes involved;
M: metastases.
Screening: Digital rectal examination and PSA-levels are used in the USA. The evidence for widespread screening is limited.

MANAGEMENT

Multidisciplinary discussion: On tumour staging and optimal treatment modality considering patients' age, comorbidity and wishes.

Low risk	<10 ng/ml and ≤6 Gleason score and <T2a stage
Intermediate risk	10–20 ng/ml or 7 Gleason score or T2b stage
High risk	>20 ng/ml or 8–10 Gleason score and >T3 stage

Active surveillance: Watchful waiting and PSA monitoring is usually the most appropriate option in low- and intermediate-risk patients.

Radical prostatectomy: For tumours localised to the gland. This can be done by either retropubic (for pelvic lymph node sampling) or perineal approach. By open surgery, laparoscopic or robotic-assisted methods.

Medical hormone therapy: LHRH analogues (e.g. goserelin) combined initially with anti-androgen (cyproterone acetate) to prevent testosterone flare. Other therapies include anti-androgens: nonsteroidal, e.g. bicalutamide, flutamide, or steroidal. Can be used as neoadjuvant therapy.

Androgen ablation surgery: Bilateral orchidectomy can slow disease progression.

Chemotherapy: Docetaxel may be used for hormone-refractory disease.

Radiotherapy: Adjuvant radiotherapy if the surgical excision margins are inadequate or if there is lymph node involvement to tumours confined to the pelvis. Brachytherapy can also be used. Neoadjuvant hormone treatment has been shown to be effective prior to external beam radiotherapy to large but localised tumours. Palliative radiotherapy can be used for bone pain and neurological complications.

COMPLICATIONS

Spread: Local growth into seminal vesicles, bladder and rectum; lymphatic spread to iliac and para-aortic nodes; blood-borne spread most commonly to bone (especially to the spine) as well as lung or liver.

From disease: Obstructive hydronephrosis, hypercalcaemia, metastatic disease.

From surgery: Impotence, urinary incontinence, urethral stricture.

From radiotherapy: Bowel and bladder damage.

From hormone therapy: Androgen deficiency can cause impotence, ↓ libido, gynaecomastia, hot flushes and osteoporosis. Tumour hormone escape (resistance to anti-androgen therapy).

PROGNOSIS

Untreated 5-year survival of 80%; radical treatment has a 10-year survival of more than 80%. Metastatic disease has a median survival of 18–24 months.

Renal carcinoma

DEFINITION
Malignancy arising from renal tubular epithelium.

AETIOLOGY
Sporadic and hereditary forms are associated with mutations in the tumour suppressor genes (*VHL*, *TSC*) or oncogene (*MET*).
Hereditary syndromes: von Hippel–Lindau disease, hereditary papillary renal carcinoma, familial renal oncocytoma and hereditary renal carcinoma. Please see **Associations/Risk Factors**.

ASSOCIATIONS/RISK FACTORS
Smoking, obesity, tuberous sclerosis, acquired cystic disease of the kidney (chronic dialysis).

EPIDEMIOLOGY
Uncommon ($\sim$3% of all adult malignancies). Male: female is 3:2. Increases with age; 75% occur in men over 60 years.

HISTORY
Often asymptomatic (90%), incidental finding during scanning. The classic triad of haematuria, flank pain and abdominal mass (only 10% patients).
Systemic signs of malignancy: Weight loss, malaise, paraneoplastic syndromes: pyrexia of unknown origin, symptoms of hypercalcaemia or polycythaemia.

EXAMINATION
May be no signs, hypertension, plethora or anaemia. Palpable renal mass. A left-sided tumour extending into the left renal vein can obstruct the left testicular vein causing a left-sided varicocoele. One-third have metastases on presentation.

INVESTIGATIONS
Urine: Dipstick (to detect haematuria), cytology.
Blood: FBC, U&Es, Ca^{2+}, LFTs (associated with paraneoplastic syndromes of hypercalcaemia, polycythaemia, abnormal LFTs in the absence of liver metastases, Stauffer syndrome), ↑ ESR in 75%.
Imaging: Ultrasound, CT or MRI scans; bone and PET scanning for metastases.
Pathology: Histological types include clear cell, chromophilic, chromophobic, oncocytoma and collecting duct.
Robson staging: I: tumour within kidney capsule. II: invades perinephric fat but not Gerota's fascia. III: invades renal vein, IVC or regional lymph nodes. IV: invades adjacent viscera or distant metastases.

MANAGEMENT
Surgery: Radical nephrectomy is the standard treatment with resection of perinephric fat, Gerota's fascia, ipsilateral adrenal gland and regional lymphadenectomy. Can be performed by transperitoneal, flank, thoraco-abdominal or laparoscopic approaches.
Radiotherapy and chemotherapy: RCC is notoriously resistant to chemotherapeutic agents (mediated by multidrug resistance p-glycoprotein). Good responses are possible with newer multikinase inhibitors such as sorafenib, sunitinib. Radiotherapy may be used for metastatic lesions.

COMPLICATIONS
Distant metastases (50% affect the lung, 33% the bone). Local invasion (e.g. IVC obstruction, invasion of perinephric fat). Local haemorrhage, clot colic. Paraneoplastic syndromes.

PROGNOSIS
Depends on type and stage of tumour. Following resection of stage I disease 5-year survival is 94%, with nodal spread 18–30% and 0–20% with distant metastases.

Testicular cancer

DEFINITION
Malignancy arising in the testes.

AETIOLOGY
Please see **Associations/Risk Factors**.

ASSOCIATIONS/RISK FACTORS
Testicular maldescent or ectopic testis ↑ risk 40 times. Others are contralateral testicular tumour, family history, mumps and maternal oestrogen exposure. Genetic changes found include amplifications and deletions in chromosome 12, and KIT gene mutations.

EPIDEMIOLOGY
Uncommon, ~1% of male malignancies, but most common malignancy in 18–35 years, trimodal peak incidence, infancy, 25–40 years and 60 years. Caucasians at a higher risk than Asian/African ethnicity.

HISTORY
Testicular lump noticed. Rarely backache due to para-aortic lymphadenopathy or shortness of breath, cough or haemoptysis from lung metastases.

EXAMINATION
Painless hard testicular mass (there may be a secondary hydrocoele). Lymphadenopathy (e.g. supraclavicular, para-aortic). Signs of pleural effusion. Gynaecomastia (resulting from HCG production).

PATHOLOGY/PATHOGENESIS
Germ cell tumours are classified as seminomas (40%, peak in 30–40 years) and nonseminomatous germ-cell tumours (60%, peak in 20–30 years), which include embryonal cell carcinoma, choriocarcinoma, yolk sac tumours and teratomas. Rarer non-germ cell tumours include Sertoli and Leydig cell tumours and non-Hodgkin's lymphoma. Seminomas are pale, cream-white, solid and well circumscribed. Teratomas are cystic in appearance with haemorrhagic and necrotic areas. **Micro**: Seminomas contain sheets of uniform, tightly packed cells that vary from well-differentiated spermatocytes to anaplastic. Teratomas can contain tissue from yolk sac, trophoblastic and embryonal cell elements with varying differentiation, and are classified based on the relative proportions.

INVESTIGATIONS
Bloods: FBC, U&Es, LFTs, tumour markers α-fetoprotein, β-HCG, LDH.
Urine: *Pregnancy test*: Positive if the tumour produces β-HCG.
Testicular ultrasound: To view primary tumour.
Staging: CT scan (abdomen, chest, brain if extensive disease). MRI in equivocal lesions or FDG-PET to evaluate residual seminoma masses. TNM staging is used or Royal Marsden Hospital staging: I – Limited to testis. II – abdominal lymphadenopathy; A: <2 cm; B: 2–5 cm; C: >5 cm. III – Nodal involvement above the diaphragm; A, B, C as above. IV – Extralymphatic metastases.

MANAGEMENT
Depends on the pathology, staging and prognostic grouping of the tumour. Patients should be offered sperm banking prior to chemo/radiotherapy.
Seminoma: Radical inguinal orchidectomy to remove the affected testis. Stage I: Options include adjuvant radiotherapy (seminomas are very radiosensitive), chemotherapy (one cycle of carboplatin) or surveillance. Stage IIA, IIB: Radiotherapy, chemotherapy or combination. Stage IIC and above: Multiagent chemotherapy, e.g. BEP (bleomycin, etoposide, cisplatin).
Nonseminomatous GCT: Radical inguinal orchidectomy. Stage I: 30% will have microscopic metastases to retroperitoneal lymph nodes. Options are surveillance or chemotherapy or primary retroperitoneal lymph node dissection (RPLND).

Testicular cancer (continued)

Stage II–IV: RPLND and/or multiagent platinum-based chemotherapy (residual retroperitoneal lymph node masses should be removed if ≥ 1 cm, as they may contain residual tumour).

COMPLICATIONS

Of disease: Metastases causing pulmonary or neurological complications.

Of treatment: *Surgery:* wound infection, nerve injury, haematoma.

Chemotherapy: Infertility, nausea and vomiting, bone marrow depression. Bleomycin can cause rashes, pneumonitis or fibrosis; platinum agents are neuro- and nephrotoxic. With long-term survival secondary malignancies and cardiac disease.

Spread: Local spread to tunica vaginalis and along the spermatic cord; lymphatic spread to para-aortic nodes, then to mediastinal and supraclavicular nodes; blood-borne spread to lungs, brain, bone and liver.

PROGNOSIS

Good with cure rates of 90–100% in early-stage disease. Seminomas are highly curable. Choriocarcinomas have the worst prognosis.

Testicular torsion

DEFINITION

A surgical emergency: twisting or torsion of the spermatic cord that results initially in venous outflow obstruction from the testis, progressing to arterial occlusion and testicular infarction if not corrected.

AETIOLOGY

Intravaginal (most common type): A high investment of the tunica vaginalis around the spermatic cord enables the testis to twist within the vaginalis.

Extravaginal (seen in neonates): When the entire testes and tunica vaginalis twist in a vertical axis on the spermatic cord (due to incomplete fixation of the gubernaculum to the scrotal wall allowing free rotation).

ASSOCIATIONS/RISK FACTORS

Imperfectly descended testes, high investment of the tunica vaginalis (bell clapper testes), long epididymal mesentery.

EPIDEMIOLOGY

Annual incidence ~1/4000. Most common cause of acute scrotal pain in 10–18-year-olds (intravaginal). Rarely occurring in neonates (extravaginal torsion).

HISTORY

Sudden-onset severe hemiscrotal pain that may be associated with abdominal pain, nausea and vomiting. The pain may awake patient from sleep, or there may be history of a similar pain that spontaneously resolved.

EXAMINATION

The scrotum on the affected side may be swollen and erythematous with a very tender swollen testis lying higher than the contralateral side and may be horizontal; a thickened cord may be palpable and the epididymis may be found to lie anteriorly. The cremasteric reflex may be absent.

Differential diagnosis: Testicular appendix torsion (appendix testes, appendix epididymis, hydatid of Morgagni): There may be a visible lesion on transillumination (blue dot sign). Epididymo-orchitis and incarcerated inguinal hernia.

PATHOLOGY/PATHOGENESIS

Twisting results in compression of the veins of the pampiniform plexus from the testis and venous congestion, with progressive ischaemia and infarction if the blood supply is not restored by detorsion.

INVESTIGATIONS

In general, an acutely tender and swollen testis in a young boy or adolescent should be considered torsion until proven otherwise and urgent exploration is required.

Doppler or duplex imaging of the testis: May be performed but should not delay surgery. Arterial inflow may be ↓ in cases of torsion and ↑ in epididymo-orchitis.

MANAGEMENT

Surgical: Exploration of the scrotum should be performed ideally within 6 h of symptoms. Consent should include counselling about bilateral orchidopexy and orchidectomy. A horizontal or midline raphe incision is made through the skin and dartos muscle. The tunica vaginalis is opened and the testis is delivered and inspected. The testis is untwisted and allowed to reperfuse, covering with a warm saline-soaked swab for a few minutes. This is followed by bilateral orchidopexy. Classically three-point fixation of testis with nonabsorbable sutures to the scrotal tissues to prevent recurrence. If the testis is found to be necrotic, orchidectomy is performed.

Testicular torsion (continued)

COMPLICATIONS

Testicular infarction and atrophy if not treated promptly. If left, the testes may become infected or impair fertility by promoting formation of anti-sperm antibodies.

Of surgery: haematoma, infection.

PROGNOSIS

From onset of pain, a testicular torsion may only survive 4–6 h. With prompt exploration most cases can be salvaged.

Urinary tract calculi

DEFINITION
Stone deposition within the urinary tract. Also known as nephrolithiasis.

AETIOLOGY
Calculi are formed by the supersaturation of urine by stone-forming compounds allowing crystallisation around a focus.

Type of calculi	Description
Calcium phosphate and calcium oxalate	80%. Can be spiculated, mulberry or dotted types
Magnesium ammonium phosphate (struvite)	10–20%. Associated with urea-splitting bacteria, e.g. *Proteus*, *Pseudomonas*, *Klebsiella*. May form 'staghorn' stones within the kidneys
Urate	Uncommon (~5%). Occurs in acidic urine, associated with gout, small bowel disease, cell lysis
Cystine	Uncommon (~1%). Forms in cystinuria, rare autosomal recessive metabolic disorder

Metabolic: Hypercalciuria, hyperuricaemia, hypercystinuria, hyperoxaluria.
Infection: Hyperuricaemia – urea-splitting bacteria.
Anatomic factors: Horseshoe kidney, caliceal diverticulae causing urinary stasis.
Kidney disease: Adult polycystic kidney disease, medullary sponge kidney, renal tubular acidosis type I.
Drugs: For example, indinavir.

EPIDEMIOLOGY
Common, prevalence: 2–3%. Lifetime risk is 5–15%. Fifteen per cent are bilateral. Male: female ratio of 3:1.

HISTORY
Can be asymptomatic. Ureteric stones can cause severe 'loin to groin' flank pain that may be associated with nausea and vomiting.
Urinary urgency, frequency, infections or retention.
Haematuria – microscopic or frank (may be absent in up to 10%).

EXAMINATION
Loin or lower abdominal tenderness. A leaking AAA is the most important differential diagnosis to consider in older patients. Signs of systemic sepsis if there is obstruction and infection.

INVESTIGATIONS
Blood: FBC, U&E (to assess renal function), Ca^{2+}, urate, PO_4^{3-}.
Urine: Dipstick, microscopy, culture and sensitivity, 24-hour urine collection.
Radiograph (KUB film): Ninety per cent of stones are radio-opaque and will show up on a plain radiograph.
Intravenous urogram: With obstructing ureteric stone, initially a delayed dense nephrogram; later films show a dilated pelvicaliceal system and a standing column of contrast down to the site of the stone (see Fig. 31).
Non-contrast CT: Most sensitive for stone detection, higher radiation dose.
Ultrasound: Can show ureteral dilation or hydronephrosis from obstructive uropathy, not sensitive for smaller stones. Used in patients with contraindications to radiation or contrast exposure, e.g. pregnancy.
Isotope renography (e.g. with DTPA or DMSA): Assessment of kidney function in complex stone disease.

Urinary tract calculi (continued)

MANAGEMENT

Acute presentation: Analgesia, fluid replacement (oral or IV). Urine collection to retrieve calculi passed for analysis. Suitable for stones not causing obstruction; majority <5 mm will pass. Alpha-blockers (e.g. alfusozin) can help stones pass by ureteric relaxation. An obstructed infected kidney should be treated as an emergency with urgent relief of obstruction, e.g. by ureteroscopy and stent or radiologically guided percutaneous nephrostomy with antibiotic and supportive measures.

Removal of calculi: Indicated if obstructing stone, continuing pain or pyrexia.

Ureteroscopy: Flexible or rigid ureteroscope is passed into the bladder and up the ureter to visualise the stone with removal by a basket, grasper or broken up with laser, ultrasound. If the stone is impacted and cannot be removed, a JJ stent should be placed to ensure urine drainage.

Extracorporeal shock-wave lithotripsy: Non-invasive. An electromagnetic or piezoelectric shock wave is focused onto calculus to break it up into smaller fragments that can pass spontaneously. Suitable for stones <2 cm as long as no obstruction to drainage.

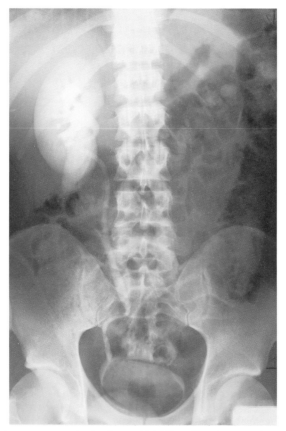

Figure 31 Intravenous urogram showing obstructed right kidney with nephrogram and a standing column of contrast down to the vesicoureteric junction.

Percutaneous nephrolithotomy: Performed for large complex stones, e.g. staghorn calculi. Following creation of a nephrostomy tract, a nephroscope is introduced and allows disintegration and removal of stones. A nephrostomy tube is left in situ for 1–2 days post op, with a nephrostogram performed to ensure stone removal and confirm ureteric drainage.

Open nephro-, pyelo- or ureterolithotomy: Rarely performed (for complex cases).

Nephrectomy: may be indicated in a non-functioning kidney.

Treatment of cause: Depends on the cause, e.g. parathyroidectomy, dietary calcium or oxalate restriction, allopurinol. Urine alkalinisation with oral potassium citrate is useful in dissolving urate and cystine stones.

Advice: Encourage high oral fluid intake.

COMPLICATIONS

Of stones: Infection, especially pyelonephritis, septicaemia, urinary retention.

Of ureteroscopy: Perforation, false passage.

Of lithotripsy: Pain, haematuria, steinstrasse (ureteric obstruction caused by a column of stone fragments).

PROGNOSIS

Good, but can be a recurrent problem (rate 50% over 5 years) and infection can potentially lead to irreversible renal scarring.

Aortic aneurysm, abdominal

DEFINITION
An abnormal localised dilatation of the abdominal aorta >3 cm (or 50% over normal diameter). Most commonly, affects the infrarenal aorta (95%), with iliac involvement in 30% (Fig. 32).

AETIOLOGY
The likely cause is collagen and elastin degeneration in the arterial wall. Often associated with atherosclerosis. Other: inflammatory (chronic inflammatory infiltrate in the vessel wall), traumatic, infective (mycotic), arteritis, connective tissue diseases e.g. Marfan's syndrome and Ehlers–Danlos type IV.

ASSOCIATIONS/RISK FACTORS
Smoking, family history (10-fold ↑ risk if first-degree relative affected), hypertension, coronary artery disease and popliteal artery aneurysms. The risk of rupture is related to diameter (Laplace's law: tension α radius, pressure). AAAs 5–5.9 cm risk 3.3% per year, 6–6.9 cm risk 9.4% per year, 7–7.9 cm risk 24% per year.

EPIDEMIOLOGY
Five percent of the population >60 years and 15% >80 years will have an AAA. Four to six times more common in men; ~6000 deaths/year in England and Wales.

HISTORY
Often asymptomatic, may be found incidentally on examination, imaging or screening.

Symptoms: Most common presentation is with rupture of an undiagnosed AAA with epigastric or back pain or collapse. Those reaching hospital usually have a leak tamponaded within the retroperitoneum.

Maybe misdiagnosed as renal colic, musculoskeletal back pain or diverticulitis. Intact aneurysms may cause back pain due to vertebral erosion or lower limb ischaemia due to distal embolisation. Rarely, present with massive GI bleeding due to erosion into the duodenum or high-output cardiac failure due to aortocaval fistula.

EXAMINATION
A pulsatile mass is felt above the umbilicus. If leaking or rupture, abdominal and back tenderness with pallor, tachycardia, hypotension and hypovolaemic shock, occasionally flank bruising, signs of emboli to feet.

INVESTIGATIONS
Acute presentation: Bloods: FBC, U&Es, clotting, urgent cross-matching of blood, ECG and CXR.

Bedside ultrasound: To confirm the presence and size of the aneurysm.

In stable or diagnostic uncertainty: If stable or diagnostic uncertainty.

CT scanning: Not if unstable, should go straight to theatre/endovascular suite for repair. A number of centres offer emergency EVAR.

Screening: Studies, e.g. the Multicentre Aneurysm Screening Study (MASS), have shown that screening men aged 65 years by ultrasound reduces aneurysm-related mortality, is cost effective and over a 20-year period will reduce the need for emergency surgery by more than two-thirds.

CT or MR angiography: To delineate aneurysm morphology prior to treatment.

MANAGEMENT
Conservative: UK Small Aneurysm Study demonstrated that asymptomatic aneurysms (<5.5 cm) should be managed conservatively with regular follow-up by ultrasound (3–4 cm yearly, or 6-monthly if enlargement >10% per year, 4–5.5 cm 3–6-monthly scanning) and management of cardiovascular risk factors.

Aortic aneurysm, abdominal (continued)

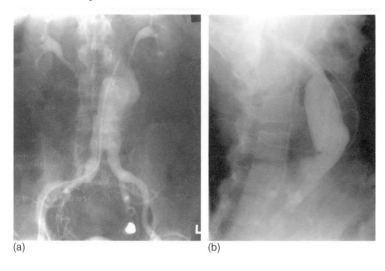

(a)

(b)

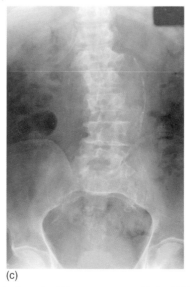

(c)

Figure 32 Plain abdominal radiographs with intravenous contrast (a) AP and (b) lateral, which demonstrate abdominal aortic aneurysms; (c) with obvious calcification in the arterial walls.

Radiological: Endovascular treatment by stent placement (EVAR) is increasing with trials underway to compare with standard open repairs. Forty to 60% of AAAs are suitable, i.e. have a satisfactory 'neck' and 'landing sites' for the endograft.

- EVAR1 compared EVAR and open surgery in patients fit for surgery and showed a 3% better aneurysm-related survival with EVAR at 4 years.
- EVAR2 compared EVAR to no intervention in unfit patients and found no differences in all-cause mortality.

Surgical: With tube or bifurcation grafts (see *Procedures*) indicated for:
- emergency treatment (e.g. suspected leaking or ruptured aneurysm);
- asymptomatic aneurysms >5.5 cm in diameter;
- symptomatic or rapidly expanding aneurysms.

COMPLICATIONS

Rupture (most frequent), distal embolus, sudden complete thrombosis, infection (gram-negative organisms or staphylococci), chronic consumptive coagulopathy, gut ischaemia, aortic-intestinal fistula, arteriovenous fistula from aneurysm eroding into the IVC.

Of surgery: Haemorrhage, graft infection, thrombosis, embolism, colonic ischaemia, renal failure, cardiac/respiratory complications and death.

Of EVAR: Above; also migration, endoleak, kinking/distortion, stent fracture, renal infarction, limb/pelvic ischaemia.

PROGNOSIS

Less than fifty per cent of patients with a ruptured AAA reach hospital alive and only about 50% of these survive (overall 80% mortality).

Elective open surgery mortality is <5% in specialist centres. EVAR has a lower mortality (~2%); however, surveillance is required and re-intervention rates are higher.

Aortic dissection

DEFINITION

A condition where a tear in the aortic intima allows blood to surge into the aortic wall, causing a split between the inner and outer tunica media, and creating a false lumen.

AETIOLOGY

Degenerative changes in the smooth muscle of the aortic media are the predisposing event. Common causes and predisposing factors:

- hypertension;
- aortic atherosclerosis;
- connective tissue disease (e.g. SLE, Marfan's, Ehlers–Danlos);
- congenital cardiac abnormalities (e.g. aortic coarctation);
- aortitis (e.g. Takayasu's aortitis, tertiary syphilis);
- iatrogenic (e.g. during angiography or angioplasty);
- trauma;
- crack cocaine.

Stanford classification divides dissection into (Fig. 33):

Type A: Ascending aorta tear (most common);

Type B: Descending aorta tear distal to the left subclavian artery.

Expansion of the false aneurysm may obstruct the subclavian, carotid, coeliac or renal arteries.

EPIDEMIOLOGY

Most common between 40 and 60 years. Males > Females.

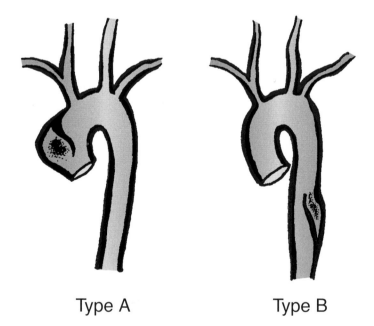

Type A   Type B

Figure 33 (Left) Stanford type A aortic dissection; (right) Stanford type B aortic dissection.

Aortic dissection (continued)

HISTORY

Sudden central 'tearing' pain, may radiate to the back (may mimic an MI).

Aortic dissection can lead to occlusion of the aorta and its branches.

Carotid obstruction: hemiparesis, dysphasia, blackout.

Coronary artery obstruction: chest pain (angina or MI).

Subclavian obstruction: ataxia, loss of consciousness.

Anterior spinal artery: paraplegia.

Coeliac obstruction: severe abdominal pain (ischaemic bowel).

Renal artery obstruction: anuria, renal failure.

EXAMINATION

Murmur on the back below left scapula, descending to abdomen.

Blood pressure: Hypertension (BP discrepancy between arms of >20 mmHg), wide pulse pressure. If hypotensive may signify tamponade, check for pulsus paradoxus.

Aortic insufficiency: Collapsing pulse, early diastolic murmur over aortic area.

Unequal arm pulses.

INVESTIGATIONS

Bloods: FBC, cross-match, U&E (renal function), clotting.

CXR: Widened mediastinum, localised bulge in the aortic arch.

ECG: Often normal. Signs of left ventricular hypertrophy or inferior MI if dissection compromises the ostia of the right coronary artery.

CT thorax abdomen: False lumen of dissection can be visualised.

Echocardiography: Trans-oesophageal is highly specific.

Cardiac catheterisation and aortography.

MANAGEMENT

Acute: If suspected, urgent CT should be performed concurrent to resuscitation. Resuscitate and monitor pulse and BP in both arms, central venous pressure, urinary catheter. Best managed in ITU setting.

Type A dissection: Treated surgically. Emergency surgery because of the risk of cardiac tamponade. Affected aorta is replaced by a tube graft. Aortic valve may also be replaced.

Type B dissection: Can be treated medically, surgically or by endovascular stenting. Control BP and prevent further dissection with IV nitroprusside and/or IV labetalol (use calcium-channel blocker if β-blocker contraindicated). Surgical repair may be appropriate for patients with intractable or recurrent pain, aortic expansion, end-organ ischemia or progression of dissection. Endovascular repair is a newer technique using endovascular stents and is available in some centres (ADSORB trial results pending).

COMPLICATIONS

Aortic rupture, cardiac tamponade, pulmonary oedema, MI, syncope, cerebrovascular, renal, mesenteric or spinal ischaemia.

PROGNOSIS

Untreated mortality: 30% at 24 hours, 75% at 2 weeks.

Operative mortality of 5–10%. A further 10% have neurological sequelae.

Prognosis for type B better than type A.

Arteriovenous fistulae and malformations

DEFINITION

Arteriovenous fistula: An abnormal communication between an artery and vein that bypasses the capillary bed.

Arteriovenous malformations: Malformation with normal endothelium.

Haemangioma/angioma: Malformation with endothelial hyperplasia.

AETIOLOGY

Congenital: Divided into haemangiomas, (e.g. strawberry naevi) and malformations (AVMs). The latter is divided into low flow or high flow (e.g. hepatic or pulmonary AVM; Fig. 34(a)).

Hereditary: AVMs and haemangiomas are associated with many different hereditary syndromes, e.g. Klippel–Trénaunay, Kasabach–Merritt, Sturge–Weber, von Hippel–Lindau and hereditary haemorrhagic telangiectasia (Osler-Weber-Rendu syndrome).

Acquired: Trauma, tumours (e.g. glomus tumour, hypernephroma and sarcomas), infection, inflammation (e.g. aorto-venocaval fistula) or iatrogenic (e.g. Brescia–Cimino fistula for haemodialysis or portocaval shunt in portal hypertension; Fig. 34(b)).

EPIDEMIOLOGY

Cutaneous haemangiomas are very common, the others less so.

HISTORY

Presentation is variable, depending on the site and size of the AVM and symptoms may be due to local or systemic effects (see *Complications*).

Congenital cutaneous haemangiomas are often visible from or soon after birth.

Malformations usually grow with age, puberty or pregnancy.

Those within internal organs may only be detected once complications develop.

Other presentations include varicose veins, limb swelling or pain.

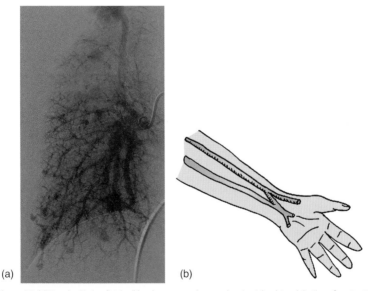

(a)   (b)

Figure 34 (a) Brescia–Cimino fistula; (b) pulmonary angiogram showing 'clouds' on injection of contrast into pulmonary artery indicating pulmonary AVMs. There is also a large AVM in the superior lobe.

EXAMINATION

Cutaneous haemangiomas (Campbell de Morgan spots) are usually scarlet in colour, firm and cannot be emptied of blood on compression.

Internal AVMs may be revealed by an overlying bruit or palpable thrill, possibly with reduced distal pulses and ↑ pulse pressure.

Signs of complications (see *Complications*).

INVESTIGATIONS

Imaging of AVMs: Depends on the site of the lesion. Modalities used include duplex scanning, CT or MRI scanning or invasive angiography.

SPECT scan: Quantification of AV shunting uses radiolabelled microspheres which are introduced into an artery and are too large to pass through capillaries. Those passing through AVMs are trapped in the lungs and quantified using gamma camera.

MANAGEMENT

Conservative: Cutaneous haemangiomas usually undergo spontaneous regression by the end of the first year of life. Internal organ AVMs may not necessitate treatment and can be monitored.

Interventional radiology: In the case of internal AVMs or fistulae, embolisation with metal coils, tissue adhesive or particles can be performed.

Surgery: Often difficult, but excision (after pre-operative embolisation) may be possible in the case of small and accessible AVMs.

Stereotactic radiosurgery: Useful on small AVMs, may take years for full effect.

COMPLICATIONS

Cutaneous: Cosmetic disfigurement, ulceration, bleeding.

Organ-specific: E.g. brain AVMs can cause focal neurological deficits, seizures or stroke; pulmonary AVMs can cause haemoptysis or parodoxical embolism.

Distal: Ischaemia of peripheral tissues.

Systemic: High-output cardiac failure in the case of large AVMs.

PROGNOSIS

Depends on site and aetiology. Ninety per cent of haemangiomas regress by 5–10 years; 1–4% annual risk of haemorrhage in cerebral AVMs.

Carotid artery disease (atherosclerosis)

DEFINITION

Narrowing of the carotid artery by atherosclerosis; a common cause of stroke.

AETIOLOGY

Atheromatous plaque at the common carotid bifurcation or any of the carotid branches can cause stroke or blindness by distal embolisation, thrombosis or low flow. The carotid artery bifurcation is an area of the vascular tree where atherosclerosis is common. In combination with systemic risk factors, local haemodynamics, including low shear stress and ↑ turbulence affecting the outer walls opposite the flow divider, predispose to atheroma development, luminal narrowing and risk of plaque rupture, thrombosis or embolism.

EPIDEMIOLOGY

Common, third leading cause of death in the UK and major cause of long-term disability, ↑ incidence with age, more common in men.

HISTORY

Often asymptomatic.

Amaurosis fugax: Transient unilateral vision loss – 'like a curtain coming down' caused by embolism into the ophthalmic artery (internal carotid artery branch).

Transient ischaemic attacks (TIA): Focal symptoms lasting <24 hours, may be a precursor of a stroke. The ABCD2 score (below) helps identify patients at high risk of stroke following TIA (≥4 needs investigation and treatment in 24 hours):

ABCD2 factor	Points
Age >59 years	1
BP on presentation ≥140/90	1
Clinical features	
Speech disturbance but no weakness	1
Unilateral weakness	2
Duration (minutes)	
10–59	1
≥60	2
Diabetes	1

Crescendo TIAs: TIAs that increase in duration, severity or frequency. This is associated with a critical stenosis of the internal carotid artery.

Stroke: Persistent neurological deficit (dependent on region affected by infarct).

EXAMINATION

If asymptomatic, often no abnormality on examination.

A carotid bruit, if present, does not reflect the degree of stenosis.

Signs of TIA or CVA (e.g. dysarthria, dysphasia, weakness in limbs).

INVESTIGATIONS

Duplex Doppler carotid ultrasound: Non-invasive imaging to assess degree of stenosis.

CT, CTA, MRI and MRA: Brain and carotid imaging (Fig. 35).

Angiography: Invasive (risk stroke ~1%), very accurate assessment of stenosis severity.

MANAGEMENT

The Early use of Existing Preventive Strategies for Stroke (EXPRESS) study showed that urgent assessment and treatment reduced the 90-day risk of recurrent stroke by 80%. All with TIA/minor stroke should be seen in a TIA clinic (urgency determined by ABCD2 scoring).

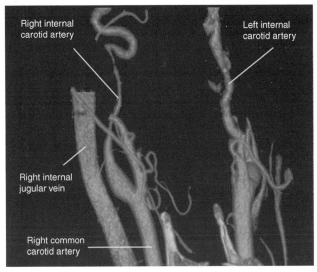

Figure 35 CT-angiogram with 3D reformatting demonstrating right internal carotid stenosis.

Medical treatment: Low-dose aspirin, stopping smoking and treatment of other risk factors, hypercholesterolaemia, hypertension and diabetes, for:
- asymptomatic stenosis,
- <70% internal carotid artery stenosis (ECST criteria), <50% (NASCET criteria), or
- inoperable disease.

Surgical treatment: Carotid endarterectomy within 2 weeks of stroke or TIA reduces risk of further stroke in ECST and NASCET trials, although carries a significant perioperative risk. May be considered in:
- symptomatic stenosis of 70–99% (ECST criteria), 50–99% (NASCET criteria), or
- crescendo TIAs not responding to medical treatment.

The role of surgical treatment in asymptomatic disease is controversial.

Angioplasty + / – stenting: Under evaluation comparing with carotid endarterectomy for symptomatic disease.

COMPLICATIONS

Complications of disease: Stroke (thromboembolic or watershed).

Complications from surgery: Cardiac ischaemia or infarction (3%), nerve injury (2–7%, mandibular branch of facial nerve, recurrent laryngeal or hypoglossal nerves), haematoma, hypertension, hypotension, perioperative stroke (1–5%). The perioperative mortality rate is 0.5–1.8%.

PROGNOSIS

For carotid artery stenosis of >70%, annual stroke rate is 10–20%.

If surgically corrected: Six- to eightfold reduction in risk of stroke compared to best medical therapy alone in patients with severe stenosis.

Carotid body tumour

DEFINITION

A tumour arising from chemoreceptor cells at the carotid bifurcation, also known as a chemodectoma.

AETIOLOGY

- Associated with mutations in subunits of the mitochondrial succinate dehydrogenase complex.
- One-third are familial with autosomal dominant inheritance (more likely to be bilateral and multiple).

Shamblin's classification:

- *Type I*: Small tumours easily dissected from carotid bifurcation.
- *Type II*: Larger more adherent, involve but do not encase vessels.
- *Type III*: Large and surrounding the carotid bifurcation.

ASSOCIATIONS/RISK FACTORS

- Associated with MEN II, NF1 and von Hippel-Lindau syndrome.
- There is an ↑ incidence in those who live at high altitudes for long periods.

EPIDEMIOLOGY

Rare. May present at any age, most commonly 50–70 years; women > men.

HISTORY

Most commonly presents as a slowly growing lump in the neck. Pressure on nearby cranial nerves may give rise to symptoms such as dysphagia, choking or hoarseness.

EXAMINATION

Neck lump in the region of the carotid triangle of the neck with transmitted pulsation. There may be evidence of cranial nerve VII, IX, X, XI paresis or palsy, Horner syndrome.

PATHOLOGY/PATHOGENESIS

Carotid body tumour is a form of paraganglioma, a tumour derived from neural crest tissue, which includes vagal body tumours, glomus jugulare tumours and pheochromocytomas. Vascular tumour with epithelioid 'chief cells' arranged in clusters or 'zellballen' surrounded by sustentacular cells. The cells are usually nonsecretory (but have the potential to secrete catecholamines).

INVESTIGATIONS

Imaging: Ultrasound, duplex scanning: Will show the relationship with the carotid bifurcation; angiography (can be CT or MR) confirms the characteristic splaying of the internal and external carotid arteries and the tumour 'blush in wine glass' appearance. CT or MRI scan: Used to determine the extent of the tumour. ^{131}I-MIBG (metaiodo-benzylguanidine) scintigraphy in functional tumours.

Direct and indirect pharyngoscopy and laryngoscopy: May be performed to assess cranial nerve involvement or pharyngeal invasion.

Urine: Urinary catecholamines, VMA, metanephrines.

MANAGEMENT

Surgery: Risk related to size/extent of tumour. As they are very vascular, pre-op embolisation of large tumours can be performed (controversial) and blood should be cross-matched preoperatively. *Surgical excision of the tumour*: Incision is based on tumour position and size. Careful dissection and control of the carotid arteries, jugular vein and identification of nerves. The tumour feeding vessels are ligated and the tumour is carefully dissected from the carotid vessels. Type II tumours often require an intraoperative shunt and replacement or sacrifice of the internal carotid artery.

Radiotherapy: For frail patients, and those with significant comorbidities or recurrent tumours.

Chemotherapy: In systemic metastases, agent used include vincristine, dacarbazine, cyclophosphamide and ^{131}I-MIBG

COMPLICATIONS

Tumour: Local invasion causing cranial nerve palsies, distal metastases.

Surgery: Bleeding, nerve injury ($\sim$15%, mandibular branch of VII, IX, X, especially the recurrent laryngeal nerves, XII), risk of stroke.

PROGNOSIS

Most are benign with 5–7% malignant, with spread to bone, liver and lung; greatest risk in young patients with heritable tumours. Characteristically slow growing; most patients can be cured by surgery.

Deep vein thrombosis

DEFINITION
Formation of a thrombus within the deep veins (most commonly of the calf or thigh).

AETIOLOGY
Virchow's triad: Venous stasis, vessel wall injury and blood hypercoagulability.

ASSOCIATIONS/RISK FACTORS
Risk factors:
Inherited: Factor V Leiden, Protein C or Protein S deficiencies, Prothrombin mutation, Antithrombin III deficiency.
Acquired: Oral contraceptive pill, surgery, immobility, obesity, pregnancy, polycythemia, anti-phospholipid syndrome, smoking, active malignancy, nephrotic syndrome, heparin-induced thrombocytopenia.

EPIDEMIOLOGY
Common, especially in hospitalised patients; exact incidence unknown. Long-term complications of DVT (venous insufficiency, ulceration) affect 0.5% population. Estimated 145 per 100,000.

HISTORY
Asymptomatic or lower limb swelling or tenderness. May present with signs/symptoms of a pulmonary embolus.

EXAMINATION
Examine for swelling, calf tenderness.
Severe leg oedema and cyanosis (phlegmasia cerulea dolens) is rare.
Respiratory examination for signs of a pulmonary embolus.

Wells Clinical Prediction Score	Score
Lower limb trauma or surgery or immobilisation in a plaster cast	+ 1
Bedridden for >3 days or surgery within the last 4 weeks	+ 1
Tenderness along deep venous system	+ 1
Entire limb swollen	+ 1
Calf >3 cm bigger circumference, 10cm below tibial tuberosity	+ 1
Pitting oedema	+ 1
Dilated collateral superficial veins (non-varicose)	+ 1
Malignancy (including treatment up to 6 months previously)	+ 1
Alternative diagnosis more likely than DVT	−2
Clinical probability of DVT	High >3
	Moderate 1–2
	Low <1

INVESTIGATIONS
Doppler ultrasound: Gold standard. Good sensitivity for femoral veins, less sensitive for calf veins.
Bloods: D-dimers (fibrinogen degradation products) are sensitive but very non-specific and only useful as a negative predictor in low-risk patients. If indicated (e.g. recurrent episodes), a thrombophilia screen should be sent, prior to starting anticoagulation. FBC (platelet count prior to starting heparin), U&E and clotting.
ECG, CXR and ABG: If there is suggestion that there might be PE.

MANAGEMENT
Anticoagulation: Patients should be treated with heparin while awaiting therapeutic INR from warfarin anticoagulation. DVTs not extending above the knee treated with anticoagulation for 3 months, while those extending beyond the knee require anticoagulation

for 6 months. Recurrent DVTs may require long-term warfarin. If active anticoagulation is contraindicated and/or high risk of embolisation, placement of an IVC filter, e.g. Greenfield filter, by interventional radiology is indicated to prevent embolus to the lungs.

Prevention: Use of graduated compression stockings. Mobilisation if possible. At-risk groups (immobilised hospital patients) should have prophylactic heparin, e.g. low-molecular-weight heparin if no contraindications.

COMPLICATIONS

Of the disease: Pulmonary embolus, damage to vein valves and chronic venous insufficiency of the lower limb (post-thrombotic syndrome). Rare: venous infarction (phlegmasia cerulea dolens).

Of the treatment: Heparin-induced thrombocytopaenia, bleeding.

PROGNOSIS

Depends on extent of DVT. Below-knee DVTs lower risk of embolus; more proximal DVTs have higher risk of propagation and embolisation, which if large, may be fatal.

Ischaemic lower limb, acute

DEFINITION
Limb ischaemia due to sudden occlusion of the supplying artery.

AETIOLOGY
Pathophysiology: Sudden interruption of blood supply. Emboli tend to lodge at sites of vessel bifurcation. There are two phases of cell injury:
• ischaemic injury as tissues are deprived of blood supply and
• reperfusion injury if blood flow is restored.
Thrombosis: Atherosclerosis, aneurysm, graft stenosis, low flow, e.g. hypovolaemia, thrombotic states.
Embolism: 90% from heart, 9% from great vessels, 1% other. Atrial fibrillation, recent MI, valvular heart disease, aneurysms, atrial myxoma.
Vascular injury: For example, trauma or dissection.

EPIDEMIOLOGY
Estimated at 14 per 100,000 incidence.

HISTORY
6 Ps: pallor, pain, paraesthesia, pulselessness, paralysis, 'perishingly' cold limb. Symptoms and signs depend on the site of occlusion, duration of ischaemia and degree of collateral circulation.
Embolus more likely if severe, sudden onset and potential source identifiable, e.g. atrial fibrillation.
Thrombosis usually if less severe (collaterals present), history of claudication or peripheral vascular disease, no obvious source of embolus.

EXAMINATION
Limb is pale with absent pulses; capillary return is slow.

Category	Description	Neurological findings	Doppler ultrasound
I	Viable	No sensory changes or weakness	Audible arterial and venous bruit
II	Threatened (marginally)	Minimal pain	Often inaudible arterial and audible venous bruit
III	Threatened (immediately)	Mild to moderate pain	Usually inaudible arterial and audible venous bruit
IV	Irreversible	Profound deficit	No signals

After several hours, there is venous stagnation with a resulting mottled appearance and fixed staining in late stages due to capillary rupture. Sensation is altered, and if ischaemia is severe, anaesthesia with muscle paralysis, signifying the limb may be nonviable.

INVESTIGATIONS
Bloods: FBC, U&Es, coagulation profile, G&S, thrombophilia screen.
Imaging: CXR, Doppler or duplex scanning of blood flow, arteriography to demonstrate the site of occlusion and plan intervention if limb viable.
ECG: Looking for atrial fibrillation.

MANAGEMENT
Immediate: ABCs, analgesia, heparin anticoagulation to prevent thrombus propagation.
Surgical: Revascularisation within 6 hours in order to salvage limb. Operative risk is often high due to underlying heart disease. Postoperative anticoagulation is essential.

If embolus: Embolectomy, which involves isolation of artery, arteriotomy and introduction of a Fogarty balloon-tipped catheter that is passed beyond the embolus, the balloon inflated and withdrawn to retrieve the embolus.

If acute or chronic thrombosis: The limb may remain viable for a longer time due to collateral formation, and percutaneous intervention is an option, e.g. aspiration, intra-arterial thrombolysis with local infusion of, e.g., t-PA, and angioplasty of underlying stenoses.

If thrombosis but the limb is not likely to remain viable for 12–24 hours necessary for this procedure: Urgent reconstructive surgery is required, if technically possible with autogenous (saphenous vein) or synthetic (e.g. PTFE or Dacron) bypass grafting. If risk of compartment syndrome, fasciotomy is required.

If nonviable limb: Limb amputation.

COMPLICATIONS

From disease: Gangrene, limb loss, death.

From intra-arterial thrombolysis: Mortality (1–2%), CVA, major haemorrhage.

Post-treatment: Reperfusion syndrome, compartment syndrome, rhabdomyolysis, rethrombosis.

PROGNOSIS

Risk of limb loss is up to 30%; mortality ~10%, with major mortality factor underlying cardiac disease.

Ischaemic lower limb, chronic

DEFINITION

Chronic arterial insufficiency to the lower limbs resulting in consequences ranging from pain on exercise (intermittent claudication) to ulceration or gangrene.

AETIOLOGY

Atherosclerosis in the lower aorta, iliac, femoral or other leg arteries.

ASSOCIATIONS/RISK FACTORS

Smoking, hypertension, diabetes, hypercholesterolaemia, family history.

EPIDEMIOLOGY

Common, prevalence 7–15% of elderly population; male: female is 2: 1. Annual incidence of critical limb ischaemia is 50–100/100,000 in the UK.

HISTORY

La Fontaine classification system of severity:
 I. Asymptomatic.
 II. Intermittent claudication. Crampy pain in the calf, coming on during exercise after a constant distance (claudication distance), relieved within a few minutes of exercise cessation.
 III. Rest pain. Severe aching pain that typically comes on in foot/lower limb at night, with some relief by hanging the leg over side of the bed.
 IV. Limb ulceration or gangrene.

Critical ischaemia: When there is rest pain >2 weeks, ulceration or gangrene, indicating severe arterial insufficiency threatening the viability of the limb.

Leriche's syndrome: When buttock and thigh claudication and impotence result from lower aortoiliac occlusion.

EXAMINATION

Examine the cardiovascular system, signs of hyperlipidaemia, carotid bruits, signs of ischaemic heart disease, abdominal aortic aneurysm.

If ischaemia is severe in lower limbs, there is shiny atrophic skin with hair loss or atrophic nails, and ulcers tend to be painful and have a 'punched-out' appearance (e.g. under toes or classically over lateral malleolus). Peripheries cool to the touch with prolonged capillary return time, weak or absent pulses. Listen for bruits.

Buerger's test: Elevation of the leg results in pallor, venous guttering, followed by dependent rubor.

Ankle-brachial pressure index (ABPI): Measured using a handheld Doppler; determined as the systolic ankle pressure divided by the brachial pressure. Normal >0.9; claudication 0.8–0.6.

Critical ischaemia: <0.5 or ankle systolic <50 mmHg or toe systolic <30 mmHg (values may be falsely high in diabetics due to poorly compressible vessels).

INVESTIGATIONS

Imaging: Arterial duplex, CT or MR angiography. Digital subtraction angiography in those having intervention.

Bloods: FBC, lipids, glucose, clotting and group and save preintervention.

MANAGEMENT

Medical: Stop smoking, encourage exercise; supervised programs have been shown to be effective. Treatment of other cardiovascular risk markers, e.g. statins, antihypertensives (avoid β-blockers), aspirin. Prostacyclin infusions are sometimes used in those with critical ischaemia unable to tolerate other interventions.

Endovascular surgery (see Procedures): Balloon angioplasty and/or stenting of arterial stenoses.

Surgical: For critical ischaemia or incapacitating intermittent claudication.

Revascularisation: Method depends on the site of occlusion.

Aortoiliac occlusive disease: Aorto-bifemoral bypass or sometimes axillo-bifemoral bypass, unilateral iliac disease (femoro-femoral or ilio-femoral bypass).

Femoropopliteal disease: Femoropopliteal, femorotibial or femorodistal bypass grafting using autogenous, e.g. saphenous vein (either reversed or *in situ* with valves destroyed with valvulotome) or synthetic grafts, e.g. PTFE. With the latter, a vein patch (Millar cuff) at the distal anastomosis significantly improves longer-term patency rates. Post-op surveillance of the graft by duplex scanning.

Amputation: Indicated for end-stage atherosclerotic disease, if revascularisation is technically impossible or there is significant necrosis or spreading sepsis. Revascularisation may enable below-knee amputation rather than above-knee; the former is associated with better post-op mobility and prosthetic limb use.

COMPLICATIONS

Pain, ulceration, gangrene, if wet, risk of systemic sepsis and multiorgan dysfunction.

From angioplasty: 3–4% risk, e.g. groin haematoma, thrombosis, embolism, dissection, flap, failure.

From bypass grafting:

- *Early*: Cardiac events, graft thrombosis, haemorrhage, lymphocoele, oedema, infection.
- *Late*: Thrombosis, false/anastomotic aneurysm, graft stenosis. In general, patency rates above knee (70–80% at 3 years) > below knee.

PROGNOSIS

Lower limb ischaemia is a marker of atherosclerosis throughout the vascular tree and patients are at ↑ risk of MI and stroke. Approximately 40% individuals with intermittent claudication improve, 40% remain stable and 20% progress over 5 years requiring intervention.

Varicose veins

DEFINITION

Veins that have become elongated, dilated and tortuous, most commonly the superficial veins of the lower limbs. Thread veins, 'spider veins' or reticular veins refer to smaller superficial venous telangiectasias and varicosities.

AETIOLOGY

Primary: Due to genetic or developmental weakness of the vein wall resulting in ↓ elasticity, dilation over time and valvular incompetence.

Congenital conditions associated with varicose veins include Klippel-Trenaunay syndrome (port wine stains, varicose veins and associated hypertrophy limb tissue), Parkes Weber syndrome (as KT, but with arteriovenous fistulas).

Secondary: Venous outflow obstruction: Pregnancy, pelvic malignancy, ovarian cysts, ascites, lymphadenopathy, retroperitoneal fibrosis.

Valve damage: Following deep vein thrombosis (DVT). High flow: Arteriovenous fistula.

EPIDEMIOLOGY:

Common, ↑ with age; prevalence: 10–15% adult men; 20–25% adult women.

HISTORY

Patient may complain about cosmetic appearance or experience symptoms such as aching in the legs, worse towards the end of the day or after standing for long periods; swelling, itching or complications such as bleeding, infection or ulceration. Enquire about previous history of DVT, predisposing factors and vascular risk factors.

EXAMINATION

Inspection: Inspect (patient standing) for vein distribution, skin changes, e.g. varicose eczema, lipodermatosclerosis, oedema, atrophie blanche or ulceration.

Palpation: Fascial defects along the dilated veins, the sites of incompetent perforators, may be palpated. A cough impulse may be felt over the SFJ. The tap test refers to an impulse felt distally along the vein after tapping over the SFJ (normally not present due to competent valves). Presence of foot pulses should be documented. Palpation of a thrill or auscultation of a bruit suggests an AV fistula.

Trendelenburg test: Can localise sites of valvular incompetence. With the patient supine, the leg is elevated and the veins are emptied. A hand/tourniquet is used to compress the SFJ. The leg is placed in the dependent position and filling of the veins observed before or after the tourniquet/hand is released.

Hand-held Doppler: Can demonstrate the site of valvular incompetence.

Rectal or pelvic examination: May be performed if secondary causes are suspected.

PATHOLOGY/PATHOGENESIS

Theories on pathogenesis of varicose veins include primary valvular incompetence and the development of weakness of the vein wall due to abnormalities of collagen and elastin with fibrosis of the tunica media in advanced stages. Other factors, including venous hypertension and hormonal changes, are also implicated.

INVESTIGATIONS

Imaging: Duplex ultrasound: Locates sites of incompetence or reflux. Also to exclude DVT (important if surgery contemplated). Magnetic resonance venography: For complex cases.

MANAGEMENT

Conservative: Advice on exercise (improves the calf muscle pump) and elevation of the legs at rest. Class II support stockings can be used to aid venous return and reduce swelling.

Surgical: SFJ ligation, long saphenous vein stripping to the knee and avulsion of varicosities via small stab incisions are performed. The short saphenous vein is not stripped, just ligated to avoid damage to the sural nerve.

Varicose veins (continued)

Endovenous procedures: Increasingly more popular, and can be performed under local anaesthesia. Endovenous laser treatment (EVLT) is used to ablate the long saphenous vein following tumescent infiltration of local anaesthetic around the vein under ultrasound guidance. Radiofrequency ablation similarly involves thermal injury and ablation. Foam sclerotherapy involves injection of sclerosing foam along the vein under ultrasound guidance, causing endothelial damage, inflammation and subsequent fibrosis of the vein. After all treatments, the legs are bandaged and early mobilisation is encouraged.
Venous telangiectasia and reticular veins: Microinjection or laser sclerotherapy.

COMPLICATIONS

Venous pigmentation, eczema, lipodermatosclerosis, venous ulceration, superficial thrombophlebitis.
Of treatment: Recurrence. Endovenous treatment: Skin burns, nerve injury, bruising, embolism, DVT. Surgery: Haemorrhage, infection, paraesthesia or nerve injury (up to 6%).

PROGNOSIS

In general, slowly progressive. Recurrence rates post surgery can be up to 40%

Topic Index